**Supplementing y
reviews and inde
(IME's), 3rd editic
Reviews & IME's**

MW01258093

Author: Todd Finnerty
ISBN-13: 978-0-9819955-6-4
Medicine, Psychology

Todd Finnerty, Psy.D.
100 E. Campus View Blvd, suite 250
Columbus, OH 43235
e-mail: toddfinnerty@toddfinnerty.com
Phone: (330)495-8809
Twitter: @DrFinnerty

This is Your *Little Black Book* for Success in Reviews & IME's

<u>About the Directory in this Book</u>

Congratulations! You're about to save yourself countless hours of research on companies that provide referrals for records review work and IME's as well as non-clinical career opportunities; I've done that research for you. It took me years to find the companies in this book (but now we're going to find even more opportunities together).

<u>Amazon Reviews from the first edition:</u>

"Outstanding book and a tremendous resource for Clinicians! Highly recommend this thorough directory by Dr Finnerty."

"Excellent book, concise with lots of information"

About Dr. Todd Finnerty

I'm a psychologist in Columbus, Ohio. I've worked as a medical consultant performing file reviews on Social Security disability claims since 2004. I also perform IME's related to functional impairment (workers' compensation; disability) as well as other medical records file review (ex: for short term and long term disability insurance policies. You can follow me on twitter at https://twitter.com/DrFinnerty; you can learn more about me, what I do at http://www.toddfinnerty.com

Introduction

I've written this book for a few reasons: First of all, I want to support those kindred professionals who dare to do things a little bit differently and take on roles that aren't always viewed as traditional or typical. Among those roles are medical records reviews and IME's. Please note: I use the term Independent Medical Examination, "IME," broadly for this book; I know that in some jurisdictions and with some referral sources it has a specific meaning and there are other terms for evaluations that could be used for the title as well. This is a general book designed to tell you how to get these referrals (not how to do an examination for your specific specialty). I would also like to be open in the very first paragraph that I believe "independent" medical examinations and file reviews really are and should be **independent** regardless of who paid for them (unlike the spirit behind terms like "defense medical examinations" that attorneys may sometimes use). Ethically, as professionals we are tasked with offering as independent and unbiased an opinion as we can. With that out of the way let's help you find some referrals.

This book answers the question "how do I get started performing medical records reviews and/or IME's?" It doesn't answer the question academically; it gives you a directory with the specific details that are necessary to reach out to the companies you need to know to get work in this area. However, this book is not intended to be an academic treatise on forensic or medicolegal practice specific to your discipline or specialty, nor does it aim to tell you how to perform an examination within your chosen medical specialty. It is first and foremost a directory of opportunities for you to pursue. You can also look for courses related to forensic/medicolegal practice within your specialty (most of these training are unlikely to tell you the specific places to look to actually get referrals for this work-- that is the point of this directory).

This book provides resources for both professionals who are new to this area and those who are already performing these services. It gives you the actual names of referral sources that you'll need to grow your medical records review and/or IME's practice. For example, this book includes a detailed directory of hundreds of potential referral source companies and potential employers for non-clinical careers.

The referral source list will continue to expand and adapt over the years. I'm offering a give-a-referral-source and get-all-of-the-referral-sources option to help keep it growing. If you email toddfinnerty@toddfinnerty.com a referral source that isn't in the directory (and I use it for the next edition of this book) I'll send you the full, updated list of referral sources for the next edition for free as an Excel spreadsheet. This way by giving one or more referral sources you get to receive the entire list of referral sources, including all the new referral sources we discover for the next edition, for free. This will help us continue to grow the referral source list and keep it updated with new and relevant opportunities. I also sell copies of the latest Excel spreadsheet on the website http://www.ReviewsandIMEs.com.

I wrote this book with a goal of having it pay for itself. This book will help you get referrals and/or find a non-clinical career. The cost of this book is less than you'd make from just one new referral in many cases. This book is not an overly academic, theoretical treatise on file reviews and IME's--it is a practical resource directory full of specific information related to getting these opportunities. This book is an investment which will pay for itself.

In addition, if you go to the website
http://www.ReviewsandIMEs.com you can network
with our free community of physicians, psychologists,
chiropractors, and other healthcare professionals (as
well as representatives from some of these companies).
You'll also find other opportunities like listing your
practice information on online directories. There is a
weekly email newsletter you can subscribe to for free
which discusses relevant news and opportunities in
Reviews & IME's. We also maintain free networking
groups you can find here; you're invited to join us and
start networking now:

LinkedIn: https://www.linkedin.com/groups/8494036

Facebook:
https://www.facebook.com/groups/reviewsandimes
/

There are opportunities for professionals who no longer want to see patients. However, a larger number of the opportunities prefer professionals who are in at least part-time active clinical practice. For those professionals, supplementing their income with reviews and IME's can also actually help them and their patients in the treatment portion of their practice. For example, viewing the documentation of other professionals can help improve your own documentation. In addition, by performing utilization reviews and other types of file reviews for insurance companies it can help in improving your capacity to deal with insurance companies in your healthcare practice; you'll develop a better grasp of the system and what should go in your own documentation and billing practices. IME's and disability reviews can also help a professional focus on their patient's daily, real-world functional impairment and not just their reported symptoms.

Types of Opportunities
(ex: personal injury; malpractice, quality assurance, standard of care, private disability insurance claims; Social Security disability claims; Veterans' and other disability programs like state retirement programs; workers' compensation; health care utilization review; medical necessity; pre-authorization)

What types of opportunities tend to be available in records reviews and IME's? There are a wide variety. There are a number of settings where an independent evaluation (IME) or a file review may be asked for; particularly in medico-legal contexts.

For example, someone may be filing for private disability insurance benefits or Social Security disability. They may also be filing for disability through another government agency such as the VA or a public retirement system. There may be a workers' compensation claim. There could be a malpractice or personal injury legal case or an organization may have concerns about whether a professional met the standard of care for quality assurance purposes. In addition, file reviews may be requested in the context of health insurance claims. These utilization reviews may be related to preauthorization and/or whether procedures are or were medically necessary.

Typically, in contexts related to disability claims, reviewers and examiners are asked questions that assist with determining the extent of functional impairment a claimant may experience. This could be a question in workers' compensation and personal injury related claims as well, though these could also focus on whether the treatment someone is requesting is medically necessary or not. The question of medical necessity if often central to work with health insurance companies. In addition, sometimes the referral may be for quality assurance or a malpractice referral. In these instances, the questions sometimes focus on whether the provider's treatment met the standard of care and/or caused the patient's injury. The company profiles/referral source directory in this book details specific opportunities with each source.

The good news is many of these companies will provide training to new consultants who start working with them. Many — probably most-- of the companies will train you on the specifics of their program. If you see an opportunity that looks interesting reach out to the company to discuss it.

The Company Profiles/ Referral Source List
The following are companies/sources which are good prospects for you to consider for various lines of work in Reviews & IME's. Some may offer employment as a Medical Director or in-house reviewer while others may primarily refer to outside contractors. Some may only operate primarily in one state or region while others operate nationally throughout the United States. If you know of any changes or additions for this directory for the next edition please email me at toddfinnerty@toddfinnerty.com. Thank you!

###
1-888-OhioComp, inc.
1-888-OhioComp, inc. [Ohio-based; Workers Comp]
http://www.1-888-ohiocomp.com/
hr@1-888-ohiocomp.com

from their website: "1-888-OHIOCOMP proudly serves Ohio's employers and injured workers. We commit our resources and staff to provide exceptional customer service, aggressive medical case management, and quality health care focused on an early and safe return to work." They note that "1-888-OHIOCOMP aggressively manages workers' compensation claims to ensure quality, cost-effective medical treatment and return-to-work services. We serve over 46,000 employers and manage over 300,000 claims. 1-888-OHIOCOMP is a certified Ohio managed care organization serving employers and their injured workers in all 88 counties. 1-888-OHIOCOMP maintains a health-care provider network to deliver the highest quality medical care to injured workers. 1-888-OHIOCOMP Medical Case Manager program has been URAC accredited since 2002."

3-Hab [Ohio-based, Workers Comp]
3-Hab [Ohio-based, Workers Comp]
http://www.3hab.com/
       info@3hab.com

"3-HAB is a physician-directed communications link among medical providers, employers, and employees to ensure quality care to injured workers promoting rapid recovery from injuries and industrial diseases, thus permitting quick resumption of work within safe environments."

Access Medical Evaluations...
Access Medical Evaluations
P.O. Box 510837
Livonia, MI 48151
(734)425-1102
Fax (734)425-1042

AccessEvaluation@aol.com
Primarily IMEs
No known website

Accordant Health Services
Accordant Health Services
www.accordant.com
info@accordant.com

"Accordant is the recognized leader in delivering comprehensive care management services for rare diseases on behalf of our contracted clients, which include health plans, employers, and third party administrators (TPAs) for more than 19 years. Eligible members receive our services through our association with their health plan or benefit provider. Our fully integrated programs improve the quality of life for those who are ill, as well as their families and their caregivers, while significantly reducing overall health care costs for our clients. Accordant is a wholly owned subsidiary of CVS Caremark."

Accretive Health

Accretive Health [utilization review/ physician advisor]   http://www.accretivehealth.com/ https://twitter.com/accretivehealth
            contactus@accretivehealth.com

"Accretive Health was founded in 2003 as a company focused on the execution and improvement of the end-to-end healthcare revenue cycle. The healthcare industry has continued to evolve and new reimbursement models have emerged. We have continued to transition and expand our service offerings to meet the changing demands.

We develop customer value by improving operational efficiencies, reducing costs, and increasing revenue. In the industry transition to value-based reimbursement, Accretive Health has developed tools and processes, ensuring we remain your operational partner as you transition to fee-for-value reimbursement models. Our capabilities help customers optimize their revenue cycles in order to meet the demands of both fee-for-service and value-based reimbursement models.

Our initial customer base in Michigan has expanded to nearly 100 hospitals and health systems spread across the country. Many of our customers are faith-based, non-profit hospitals or teaching institutions, including many of the top-rated healthcare systems in the United States."

<u>Activehealth Management...</u>
Activehealth Management
> http://www.activehealth.com/
> http://twitter.com/ActiveHealthMgt
> info@activehealth.net

"ActiveHealth Management is a national leader in population health management and passionate about helping every person achieve his or her best health. ActiveHealth also performs utilization management services for some clients. We deliver personalized guidance through our analytics and insights, care management, health, lifestyle and wellness programs to help our customers improve quality of care, lower healthcare costs, and drive sustained member engagement and behavior change. ActiveHealth® collaborates with employers, health plans, governments and providers currently helping more than 20 million people live their healthiest lives. ActiveHealth Management is an independent subsidiary of Aetna."

<u>Advanced Medical Reviews</u>
Advanced Medical Reviews
(purchased by ExamWorks)
> http://www.admere.com/
http://twitter.com/Amr_reviews

file reviews   reviewer_relations@admere.com

"Founded in 2004, AMR is setting the industry standard in providing quality independent medical case review and utilization management services that are timely, customizable and affordable. AMR offers a single source solution for all of our clients' review and utilization management needs covering all specialties and subspecialties nationwide. Our highly trained compliance staff, in-house medical director and specialized case review nurses are bolstered by a strong quality assurance process guaranteeing the highest quality standards throughout the review process.

Our commitment is to our clients and their patients. We emphasize - throughout all the
work that we do - continuous quality improvement, innovation and client satisfaction."

"Our Physician Reviewers may perform utilization reviews for workers compensation and other types of insurers and various types of medical peer reviews for health plans and third party administrators. These types of reviews include – medical necessity, peer-to-peer reviews, guideline reviews, 1st through 3rd level appeals, and length of stay reviews."

Aetna
Aetna
http://www.aetna.com
http://twitter.com/aetna

Agate Healthcare
Agate Healthcare   http://agatehealthcare.com/

(see also Centene)

AIG
AIG
http://www.aig.com
http://twitter.com/AIGinsurance

"We're ranked as one of 10 most preferred carriers of commercial insurance, and we're the #1 commercial insurer in the U.S. and Canada. We're also the world's largest nonlife insurer by market capitalization. We're humbled to serve 98 percent of the Fortune 500, 96 percent of the Fortune 1000, and 90 percent of the Fortune Global 500.

We're a market leader in helping to secure financial futures. We're ranked as the #1 provider of fixed-rate deferred annuity sales and as one of the top providers of group retirement plans. We're a leader in personal insurance in countries around the world, and we're the choice of almost half of the Forbes 400 Richest Americans."

AIM Specialty Health...
AIM Specialty Health
         http://www.aimspecialtyhealth.com/

"AIM Specialty Health® (AIM) is a leading specialty benefits management company with more than 20 years of experience and a growing presence in the management of radiology, cardiology, oncology, sleep management, and specialty drugs. Our mission is to make healthcare services more clinically appropriate, safer and more affordable. As such, we promote the most appropriate use of specialty care services through the application of widely accepted clinical guidelines delivered via an innovative platform of technologies and services."

Aimes Enterprises, inc.
Aimes Enterprises, inc.
http://www.aimes-inc.com/
IME and file reviews
cservices@aimes-inc.com
"AIMES provides and coordinates objective, independent medical evaluations throughout the United States. This medical and legal consulting firm has paralleled their services with the growing needs of the insurance industry, self insured groups and attorneys.

AIMES offers a wide network of physicians with specialties ranging from orthopedic or chiropractic care to dermatology, from internal medicine to dentistry. And since the foundation and reputation of AIMES lies in their integrated network of board certified physicians, this consulting firm can continually excel in providing efficient, quality records combined with a professional service oriented staff.Additionally, AIMES ensures that all our affiliated specialists are knowledgeable in the rules and regulations governing the performance of Independent Medical Examinations, including HIPAA compliance.

Akeso Care Management
Akeso Care Management
http://www.akesocare.com/

Utilization review opportunities

"Akeso Care Management® (AkesoCareSM) is a URAC-accredited international health care management company specializing in the complete spectrum of domestic and international medical management services. We offer a unique blend of service components and expertise in cost containment.

When you choose AkesoCare, you receive an exceptional level of multilingual, domestic and international medical management experience, honed by providing services to our clients in over 170 countries worldwide. AkesoCare collaborates with the patient, payer and provider in evaluating and directing the delivery of medical services, resulting in greater patient satisfaction and payer cost savings."

ALARIS
ALARIS
http://alarisgroup.com/
info@alarisgroup.com
https://twitter.com/ALARISGroup

"ALARIS provides workers' compensation and disability case management services that facilitate timely communication, while reducing medical and disability costs. ALARIS also ensures the delivery of high-quality treatment so the injured party can enjoy both a positive health outcome and a successful return to work.

We offer a sophisticated case management process that aims to collaboratively determine how best to implement, coordinate, monitor and evaluate an individual's unique health needs."

AliCare Medical Management...
AliCare Medical Management
http://www.alicaremed.com/
file reviews
sales@alicaremed.com

"With over two decades of experience and over 250 clients, AliCare Medical Management is recognized as one of the premier care management organizations in the United States.

A Leader In Quality
AliCare Medical Management is an established quality leader in the health care arena. Currently, AliCare Medical Management holds four separate URAC accreditations covering Utilization Management, Case Management, 24/7 Nurse HelpLine and Independent Review services. AliCare Medical Management has been accredited since 1997. AliCare Medical Management has served as a resource and beta test site to URAC and others over the years to better understand evolving trends in the care management industry.

Garry Carneal, URAC's president and CEO from 1996 to 2005, notes that, "It was at AliCare Medical Management where I first observed an integrated care management solution which helped identify a framework to create URAC's modular approach to accreditation. AliCare Medical Management's commitment to excellence and quality is first rate."

Clinical Expertise

AliCare Medical Management is supported by a team of nurses and physicians who participate in AliCare Medical Management's network of care management services. This includes an independent review panel made up of over 200 board-certified physicians and specialists. In addition, all AliCare Medical Management nurses and case mangers carry advanced professional certifications. AliCare Medical Management uses evidence-based health risk assessments, clinical guidelines and treatment plans that factor in a wide variety of patient co-morbidities, which in turn standardize and improve care management outcomes.

24/7 Nationwide Coverage
AliCare Medical Management's care management is available on a 24/7/365 platform. AliCare Medical Management and its clinicians are licensed in all states that require licensing for our business, empowering us to offer a full range of care management services nationwide including "after hour" and "out of state" coverage for our clients.

Private Label Option

Using AliCare Medical Management's technology solutions, clients can offer AliCare Medical Management's services through their own company brands. Clients take advantage of the ability to private label AliCare Medical Management services to ensure a seamless and consistent experience for the client's members while taking advantage of AliCare Medical Management's quality-based 24/7 platform. Our flexibility in customizing services creates the opportunity for clients to collaborate with us to develop unique solutions.

Patient-Centric
AliCare Medical Management understands that a key aspect to promoting better health is engaging patients. AliCare Medical Management's patient-centric approach to care management ensures that better clinical and financial outcomes can be achieved while maintaining high levels of patient satisfaction.

Next Generation Solutions
AliCare Medical Management optimizes its care management operations through a number of best in class technology solutions including a nationally recognized care management software application and a dynamic telephone system supporting its health call center operations. These solutions allow AliCare Medical Management to leverage technology to optimize its care management services both for clients and patients.

AliCare Medical Management has teamed up with several health care experts and organizations to launch a series of exciting new enhancements to its care management programs over the coming months. AliCare Medical Management is leading the way with new complex condition management strategies, communication portals, population stratification tools, and other innovative solutions."

Here are responses they were kind enough to send to my email survey:

Is there a good contact person/department to give to physicians and/or psychologists in relation to recruitment/credentialing with your organization? Is there a desired contact method (ex: an email address or phone number) for them?

Yes, they can contact Kathleen Andrade at 603-328-6612

· Do you contract directly with psychologists and/or neuropsychologists for medical records file review work or IME's?
Yes for file reviews

· Do you work directly with psychologists and/or physicians or do you go through third party companies? If so, which companies do you tend to use?
Directly

· Do you contract directly w/ physicians for medical records file review work or IME's?
<u>Contract directly</u>

· Do you ever have any employment opportunities for psychologists and/or neuropsychologists?
<u>No</u>

· Do you ever have any employment opportunities for physicians?
<u>Yes</u>

· If you employ psychologists and/or physicians, do you allow them to work from home?
<u>Yes</u>

· Do you ever have any employment or contract opportunities for nurses in relation to file reviews and/or IME work?
<u>Yes for file review</u>

· Do you ever have any employment or contract opportunities for mental health counselors/social workers in relation to file reviews and/or IME work?
<u>No</u>

· Do any of your opportunities require the professional to be in active clinical practice and if so how do you define active clinical practice? (ex: how many hours per week? What percentage of income from direct treatment?)

<u>Yes they must be in active practice meaning they</u>
<u>see/treat patients</u>

· What opportunities, if any, do you have for professionals who are not currently in active clinical practice?
<u>If they have over 5 years clinical practice behind they,</u>
<u>they can provide UM Case Reviews</u>

· Do you contract/employ professionals nationwide or are there particular areas or regions of the country you work in; which areas of the country are you currently recruiting in?
<u>Nationwide</u>

"Alicare Medical Management(AMM) is recognized as one of the nation's premier care management organizations for over two decades. AMM facilitates optimal outcomes for patients, providers, payers and other stakeholders by offering evidenced-based and patient-centric programs. Our suite of care management solutions are innovative and dynamic interventions that control costs and improve clinical outcomes. We utilize patient engagement strategies, provider education, data analytics, highly trained medical professionals, interoperable technology applications and other resources to meet and exceed our client expectations."

<u>Allegiance (Cigna)</u>
Allegiance (Cigna)
www.askallegiance.com

inquire@askallegiance.com
"Allegiance Benefit Plan Management, Inc., develops
and administers employee benefit plans for companies,
associations and government agencies.

Our highly-trained and experienced team of claims
professionals, systems and benefits experts, nurses,
attorneys, accountants and managers all take great
pride in serving you well. While Allegiance's goal is to
provide clients with the highest level of service, we
know ultimately the products and services we
administer serve the needs of individuals and their
families. In all that we do, we realize that ours is indeed
a business benefiting people.

As a third-party administrator, we offer our clients the
flexibility to contract with multiple preferred provider
organizations, managed care organizations, physician
hospital organizations, tertiary care centers of
excellence, dental and vision plans, and stop-loss
insurance carriers."

Alliance Behavioral Healthcare...
Alliance Behavioral Healthcare
      http://www.alliancebhc.org/
      ProviderNetwork@AllianceBHC.org

"Alliance is the managed care organization, or MCO,
for public behavioral healthcare for the citizens of
Durham, Wake, Cumberland and Johnston counties in
North Carolina.

Although we do not directly provide services, our job is to ensure that individuals seeking help receive the quality services and supports they are eligible for to help them achieve their goals and live as independently as possible.

To do this, we work alongside a diverse network of over 2500 private behavioral healthcare providers."

Alliant Health Solutions...
Alliant Health Solutionshttp://www.allianthealth.org/

"Alliant Health Solutions is a family of companies that provides professional services supporting the effective administration of health care programs and funding to support health care improvement initiatives. Alliant's experience spans the full spectrum of care settings and provider types, including acute care, advanced imaging, behavioral health, dental, dialysis, home health, hospice, long-term care, physician practices, skilled nursing, hospitals and more.

Through our professional services, Alliant works with public and private partners to make health care better. Patients are the center of all our work and our drive to improve health and health care. Alliant has three primary lines of service offerings that leverage evidenced-based methods, data and technology, and clinical expertise:

Healthcare Quality Improvement: making health care safer and more effective.

Utilization Management: ensuring the right care, in the right setting for the right duration.

Program Integrity: ensuring compliance and reducing improper payment, fraud, waste and abuse."

Allied Managed Care...
Allied Managed Care
http://www.alliedmanagedcare.com/

"Based on needs and criteria you define, we provide a dedicated team of bill reviewers, nurse case managers, return to work experts, certified life care planners, ergonomic specialists, medical providers and senior managers to help ensure your injured workers receive the best possible care for your money and manage the factors that escalate loss costs."

AllMed Healthcare Management...
AllMed Healthcare Managementhttps://allmedmd.com/
https://twitter.com/allmedmd

file reviews

"Founded in 1995, AllMed Healthcare Management is an independent review organization that provides comprehensive physician review solutions to payer and provider organizations across the nation. Our team integrates with yours, with medical, copy editing and customer resources that enable you to improve both your services and business goals. Our clients include leading health plans, medical management organizations, TPAs, disability carriers, hospital groups and ambulatory surgery centers."

AllOne Health
AllOne Health
http://www.allonehealth.com/

"We help employees in global organizations operate at full capacity by coordinating medical and behavioral services while helping employers manage escalating healthcare costs."

Allscripts
Allscripts
http://www.allscripts.com/
http://twitter.com/Allscripts
employment opportunities

"Allscripts is leading the healthcare IT movement into tomorrow's value-enabled world. No other IT partner integrates your information so you can take action across care sites, care teams and even across multivendor EHR systems. Imagine the value of enabling multisite integration – without having to rip-and-replace or rework any of your systems.

Hand in hand with our clients, we're pioneering comprehensive population health solutions and integrating precision medicine across the care spectrum. We partner with you to enable smarter care delivery for healthier patients, populations and communities.

Take a closer look at Allscripts. Experience how our EHR, financial management, population health management and precision medicine solutions can give you connected information and insights like never before. It's everything you need to confidently meet your clinical, operational and business goals."

Allstate
Allstate
https://www.allstate.com/
http://twitter.com/allstate

"We help customers realize their hopes and dreams by providing the best products and services to protect them from life's uncertainties and prepare them for the future."

AMCE Physicians Group...
AMCE Physicians Group
      http://www.amcephysicians.com/
      https://twitter.com/AMCEGRP
IMEs info@amcephysicians.com

"AMCE Physicians Group provides a full range of occupational health, injury and disability physical and mental health evaluations. Our goal is to provide these examinations in a timely and superior manner. Our professional staff members, headquartered in Northern Utah, are ready to be of assistance to you, the physician, and other medical and clinical staff members as you serve the clients. Please note, your role as a physician, and other clinical professionals is for evaluation purposes only. You are not expected and will not be asked to treat the client or prescribe anything to the client. It is also not your purpose to recommend any diagnostic testing or treatments. AMCE will provide you with the educational information of orientation and training in order to complete these evaluations. As emphasized in our Mission Statement and with our commitment to superior quality assurance, we believe you will be fully empowered and ready to serve the client. Diagnostic examinations are provided for clients as part of their employment or clients who apply for federal Social Security Disability Insurance, Supplemental Security Income benefits, or Department of Social and Health Services (DSHS) Non-Grant Medical Assistance. Each company has specific guidelines. Also, specific criteria must be met to qualify for Social Security Disability Insurance Income (also known as SSDI). The surveillance of worker's health is made through various types of health examinations. The main purpose of health examinations is to assess the suitability of a worker to carry out certain jobs, to assess any health impairment which may be related to the exposure to harmful agents inherent in the work process and to identify cases of occupational diseases which may have resulted from exposures at work. The following types of health examinations are carried out either on the basis of regulations or as a part of good occupational health practice:

- Pre-assignment (pre-employment) health examinations
- Periodic health examinations
- Return to work health examinations
- General health examinations
- Health examinations at termination or after ending of service

In review, medical professionals who perform evaluations play a crucial role. We rely on you, the physician, on your unbiased and objective evaluations for the best available medical information."

American Behavioral...
American Behavioral
http://americanbehavioral.com/
http://twitter.com/AmericanBehav

"American Behavioral Benefits Managers, Inc. (American Behavioral) is a full-service behavioral health care organization providing Employee Assistance Program services, behavioral health care, pre-employment and promotional psychological testing, manager and supervisor training, and critical-incident stress management. Headquartered in Birmingham, Alabama, American Behavioral serves employees and families of client companies in all 50 states and across the globe.

Since 1990, American Behavioral has grown to manage approximately 1 million covered lives while catering to the unique needs of large corporation in diverse fields such as health care, school systems, banking, retail, high-tech industries as well as governmental and municipalities. Over the past two decades, American Behavioral has provided exceptional, high quality, personal, and cost effective, behavioral health care services to employers and their employees."

American Health Group...
American Health Group
>   http://www.americanhealthgroup.com/

"American Health Group (AHG) is an independent medical management corporation and health plan administrator. We partner with self-insured corporations and employer groups to provide successful cost containment strategies. By integrating modern medical protocols with advanced health information systems, AHG redefines the industry standard of automatically paying claims. We have proven solutions with excellent results, achieving unprecedented financial savings for our clients throughout the United States."

American Health Holding
American Health Holding
>   www.americanhealthholding.com
>   ahhinfo@ahhinc.com

Utilization Management

Advanced Radiology Scheduling Services
Case Management
Maternity Case Management
Neonatal and Pediatric Case Management
Oncology Case Management
Transplant Case Management
Pre-Admission and Post-Discharge Counseling
Population Health Management
Wellness
Performance-Based Wellness and Disease Management
Disease Management
Bariatric Care Management
Maternity Management
Medical Transportation
Onsite Medical Management
Medical Review
Independent External Review
Integrated Behavioral Health
Medical Disclosure
24/7 Physician Consultations
24/7 Nurse Line and Health Information Library
Medical Cost Containment
iSuite Medical Management Software
iSuite EZ Reports

American Medical Experts...
American Medical Experts
> http://americanmedicalexperts.com
> http://twitter.com/AmerMedicalExps
> IME and file reviews

Over the past 30 years, American Medical Experts, LLC (AME) has helped thousands of plaintiff and defense attorneys obtain valuable expert witness reports, independent medical examinations - IMEs, Life Care Plans, expert opinions in automobile accidents, workers' compensation, federal claims, disability as well as all medical malpractice and personal injury cases. We have done so by working with over 10,000 world-renowned medical experts in all specialties nationwide.

American Medical Experts is the nation's leading source of Expert Witnesses for Wrongful Death cases, Nursing Home Negligence cases, Independent Medical Examinations - IMEs, Medical Expert Witness Reports, Affidavits, Certificates of Merit, etc. (depending on your State requirements), Life Care Plans, automobile accidents cases, workers' compensation, federal claims, disability as well as all areas of medical malpractice and personal injury cases.

American Medical Forensic Specialists...
American Medical Forensic Specialists
> http://www.amfs.com/
> primarily IMEs; some file reviews
> info@amfs.com

Initial Case Review
Medical Record Indexing / Chronology
Life Care Plans
Independent Medical Examinations (IMEs)
Expert Review and Testimony

Here are responses they were kind enough to send to my email survey:

·   Is there a good contact person/department to give to physicians and/or psychologists in relation to recruitment/credentialing with your organization? Is there a desired contact method (ex: an email address or phone number) for them?

Yes, interested experts can contact us at recruiting@amfs.com or simply submit their CV for consideration via our website here - http://www.amfs.com/about/become-an-expert/ and clicking on the signup form button.

·_____Do you contract directly with psychologists and/or neuropsychologists for medical records file review work or IME's?

Yes, we do. We maintain non-exclusive agreements with all of our experts and provide administrative and other support services for them in every engagement from beginning to end. We do not charge experts to join our network.

·   Do you work directly with psychologists and/or physicians or do you go through third party companies? If so, which companies do you tend to use? We work directly with experts.

·_____Do you contract directly w/ physicians for medical records file review work or IME's?_Yes.

·   Do you ever have any employment opportunities for psychologists and/or neuropsychologists? <u>No. Only consulting/review/expert witness opportunities.</u>

·   Do you ever have any employment opportunities for physicians? <u>No. Only consulting/review/expert witness opportunities.</u>

·   If you employ psychologists and/or physicians, do you allow them to work from home? <u>All of the experts in our network perform services on their own time and from any location. Again, these are not employees though.</u>

·   Do you ever have any employment or contract opportunities for nurses in relation to file reviews and/or IME work?

<u>Yes, we have physicians, psychologists, nurses, dentists and several other types of experts in our network to whom we offer review, expert witness and other consulting opportunities.</u>

·   Do you ever have any employment or contract opportunities for mental health counselors/social workers in relation to file reviews and/or IME work?

<u>Same as above. To the extent they would be an expert consultant we would have opportunities for them.</u>

·_____Do any of your opportunities require the professional to be in active clinical practice and if so how do you define active clinical practice? (ex: how many hours per week? What percentage of income from direct treatment?)___Typically, the same definition as would be required by the jurisdiction to qualify as an expert witness

·_____What opportunities, if any, do you have for professionals who are not currently in active clinical practice? We don't really have any meaningful opportunities for non-practitioners.

·   Do you contract/employ professionals nationwide or are there particular areas or regions of the country you work in; which areas of the country are you currently recruiting in?___Nationwide

·_____Which physician specialties are you actively recruiting right now? We are always adding experts in all specialties and subspecialties to our network.

·_____Are you actively seeking psychologists or neuropsychologists right now? Same as above

·   Can you provide estimates of a typical fee range that you tend to pay to psychologists and/or physicians for medical records file review and IME work (ex: do you have a typical hourly fee or per case fee/ per report fee that you are able to share)? Hourly rates vary by specialty, level of experience, academic credentials, geographic location, etc. When an expert first joins our network, these items are reviewed and we discuss rates with them but there is no set rate as it is an individual by individual process.

·   Can you provide a brief company description that you'd like included in the book?

 AMFS is a physician founded organization that has been providing medical expert witness and consulting opportunities for more than 25 years. We've worked with thousands of physicians, psychologists, dentists, nurses, healthcare administrators and other experts since 1990. We provide administrative support to our experts with best-in-class case managers and state of the art systems allowing experts to maintain focus on their practice and not get bogged down with the administrative aspects of expert consulting work.

American Specialty Health...
American Specialty Health
        https://www.ashcompanies.com/
        http://twitter.com/ashcompanies

"American Specialty Health Incorporated (ASH) is one of the nation's premier independent and privately owned specialty health services organizations, providing physical medicine provider networks and administration, fitness center networks and exercise programs, and population health solutions for health plans, insurance carriers, and employer groups. ASH contracts with more than 140 health plans nationally and administers programs for nearly 38 million members. Operating from offices in San Diego, Calif., Southlake (Dallas), Texas, Carmel (Indianapolis), Ind., and Columbia, S.C., ASH has more than 1,200 employees. Additional products offered through ASH and its subsidiaries include Healthyroads ® , FitnessCoach ® , Active&Fit ® , Silver&Fit ® , ExerciseRewards TM and others."

AmeriHealth Administrators
AmeriHealth Administrators   www.ahatpa.com
        provrelations@ahatpa.com

The AmeriHealth Family of Companies offers a range of services for individuals and employers. From locally-focused health insurance plans to national-scale programs that assist those who need it the most, we exceed our customers' expectations through innovative health insurance and wellness solutions. Learn more about our offerings, and discover how personalized health care can make a difference.

Amerisys
Amerisys
http://www.amerisys-info.com/

amerisys-contact@amerisys-info.com

"AmeriSys is a regional managed care organization founded in 1985, which originally operated under the name of ERS until 1995. For those ten years ERS was a successful regional disability management company in Florida, Georgia, the Carolinas, and other southeastern states. ERS and its sister company ISMUS were the first integrated managed care initiatives specifically for Workers' Compensation in Florida. AmeriSys is dedicated to providing comprehensive, quality services on a national basis with attention to local service. Our medical management services are provided to self-insured employers, insurance carriers, service companies and other claims organizations.

As of April 1, 2000, AmeriSys was acquired by Brown & Brown, Inc. Our relationship with Brown & Brown provides AmeriSys with tremendous resources and economic strength, assuring that AmeriSys will be there when our client needs us.

Our organization attributes our success and growth to the retention of our customers as well as word of mouth referrals. It is the reputation of service delivery and our culture of adapting our services to meet the unique and specific needs of our customers.

The unique customer-driven culture of AmeriSys, coupled with the financial strength and resources of Brown & Brown, provides a dependable and adaptable program for our customers and clients.

The primary mission of AmeriSys is to provide high quality, professional, timely services which allows the customer to manage its disability cases in a cost effective, pro-active manner meeting both long range and short range objectives."

Ameritas
Ameritas
www.ameritas.com
http://twitter.com/ameritas

Founded in 1887, Ameritas Life and its affiliated companies – offers a wide range of insurance and financial products and services to individuals, families and businesses. These products and services include life insurance; annuities; individual disability income insurance; group dental, vision and hearing care insurance; retirement plans; investments; mutual funds; asset management and public finance.

Anthem
Anthem
www.anthem.com
http://twitter.com/AnthemInc

"With a reputation for innovation, Anthem, Inc.'s affiliates are committed to establishing a relationship with customers, physicians, hospitals and other health care clinicians as trusted partners.

Consumers want a choice of products and health care professionals, and they want more control over their health care decisions. Employers also want the maximum amount of cost control while also being sensitive to employee needs.

Anthem, Inc. affiliated health plans have created a variety of PPOs, HMOs, various hybrid and specialty products, network-based dental products and health plan services that combine the attributes consumers find attractive with effective cost control techniques. Employer groups and individual members can select from basic as well as comprehensive plans to meet their specific needs. Also available are a wide range of related specialty products and other services including flexible spending accounts and COBRA administration."

Apex Healthcare
Apex Healthcare   http://www.apexmso.com/

"Since 1996, Apex Healthcare, Inc.'s mission has been to provide cost-efficient and quality services to managed healthcare providers.

Membership Eligibility
Claims Processing
Customer Service
Provider Information
Utilization Management
Care Coordination
Medical Home
Data Management"

Applied Underwriters
Applied Underwriters
www.auw.com
customerservice@auw.com

Applied Underwriters® designs financial services and workers' compensation solutions to meet the real needs of small and mid-sized businesses nationwide. With insurance carriers rated 'A+' (Superior) by A.M. Best Company and as part of the Berkshire Hathaway family, we offer rock-solid workers' compensation coverage along with some of the hardest-working products and services available on the market today.

Arrowhead Evaluation Services
Arrowhead Evaluation Services (California)
http://arrowheadeval.com/
info@arrowheadeval.com

Ascential Care
Ascential Care
http://ascentialcare.com/
https://twitter.com/ascentialcare

"Ascential Care's team works nationally to provide leading-edge patient driven and consumer minded programs to managed care. Our staff is dedicated to meeting needs. We utilize the best practices and top notch technologies to achieve our unparalleled outcomes."

Assurant
Assurant
http://www.assuranthealth.com/

"On June 10, 2015, Assurant Health's parent company, Assurant, Inc., announced an exit from the health insurance marketplace to focus on housing and lifestyle specialty protection products and services. Assurant is winding down its major medical operations. Assurant is committed to providing a smooth process for our customers and will meet all claims and benefit commitments."

Assurity Life Insurance
Assurity Life Insurance
www.assurity.com
http://twitter.com/Assurity
claimsinfo@assurity.com
life, disability, critical illness insurance

AultComp MCO (Ohio)
AultComp MCO   https://www.aultcompmco.com/
aultcompmco@aultcompmco.com

"AultComp MCO is certified by the Ohio Bureau of Workers' Compensation as a Managed Care Organization (MCO) participating in the Health Partnership Program, a system for managing workers' compensation health care in Ohio."

Avera Health Plans
Avera Health Plans
http://www.averahealthplans.com/
http://twitter.com/averahealth

"No matter where you live across the Upper Midwest, count on Avera Health, an integrated health system based in Sioux Falls, SD, for the same top-quality health services you'd find at major medical centers and regional referral facilities.

Avera serves South Dakota and surrounding areas of Minnesota, Iowa, Nebraska and North Dakota through six regional centers in Aberdeen, Mitchell, Pierre, Sioux Falls and Yankton, SD, and Marshall, MN. We serve you through 33 hospitals, 208 primary and specialty care clinics, 40 senior living facilities in addition to home care and hospice, sports and wellness facilities, home medical equipment outlets and more."

Avysion Healthcare Services
Avysion Healthcare Services
> http://healthcare.avysion.net/
> utilization review/quality info@avysion.com

"Avysion Healthcare Services provides multidisciplinary, service-based approaches that focus on producing measurable results, improved member care quality and effective cost containment to address the healthcare services needs of our various public sector clients.

With a focus on Medicaid and DoD healthcare populations and the care organizations that provide service to them, Avysion has proven and demonstrated expertise in providing a broad range of case management, medical home redirection and other administrative healthcare solutions that produce quantified, measurable results by improving member health and reducing healthcare delivery costs.

With our extensive in-house clinical staff providing both physical and behavioral health expertise, along with software services provided by our technology division, Avysion IT, our capabilities extend across both the fee-for-service (FFS) and capitated managed care service delivery programs and systems.

With competencies in Case Management, Utilization Management and Review, Quality Reviews and Audits and Administrative Support Services and Software, Avysion understands the complexities of addressing the unique physical, behavioral and pharmaceutical health issues occurring within these populations and the methods of removing barriers to effective care delivery and medical home redirection."

AXA Assistance USA
AXA Assistance USA
http://www.axa-assistance.us/

"AXA Assistance is one of the world's leading providers of emergency response and everyday assistance. Over 50 years of experience combined with an international network of providers allow the organization to deliver innovative solutions and services in the US and around the world. AXA Assistance is part of AXA Group, the 16th largest company in the world."

Baptist Hospitals of Southeast Texas...
Baptist Hospitals of Southeast Texas
http://www.bhset.net/
http://twitter.com/bhset

"The mission of Baptist Hospitals of Southeast Texas is to provide quality healthcare and Sacred Work in a Christian environment to all who need it."

Beacon Health Options...
Beacon Health Options
https://www.beaconhealthoptions.com/
http://twitter.com/beaconhealthopt
recruiter@beaconhealthoptions.com
NetworkDevelopment@beaconhs.com

"Beacon Health Options (Beacon) combines two of the country's most prominent behavioral health companies -- Beacon Health Strategies and ValueOptions. Together we serve more than 50 million people across all 50 states and the United Kingdom."

Behavioral Health Systems...

Behavioral Health Systems

http://www.behavioralhealthsystems.com/

providerrelations@behavioralhealthsystems.com

"The BHS preferred provider network offers a continuum of care through over 11,000 providers located across the nation. This continuum includes inpatient facilities, residential treatment facilities, partial hospitalization programs, intensive outpatient programs, psychiatrists, psychologists, Master's-level counselors, therapists, clinical social workers, and community mental health centers."

Behavioral Healthcare Options...
Behavioral Healthcare Options

http://www.behavioralhealthcareoptions.com/

"Established in 1991, Behavioral Healthcare Options, Inc. (BHO) is a subsidiary of UnitedHealthcare. BHO is a leader in arranging specialized mental health, addiction treatment, employee assistance and work-life services. We promote individualized problem-focused care in the least restrictive setting for our members to ensure proper treatment and minimal disruption to work and family activities.

Our clients include self-insured employers, insurance carriers, third-party administrators and union trusts. With a willingness to customize products and services, we enable our clients to provide the best benefits for their members and/or employees. The Life Connection (TLC), our Employee Assistance Program (EAP), offers tools and resources to help employers and employees resolve issues at work and balance home and work-life. Our innovative services, comprehensive training programs, and on-going management support help our clients meet the ever-changing issues encountered in daily life."

Benchmark IME (Canada)
Benchmark IME (Canada)
http://www.benchmarkime.com/
Info@benchmarkime.com

"Wellpoint Health Services Corp. ("Wellpoint") is excited to announce a merger with Benchmark Independent Medical Examination Inc. ("Benchmark")"

BHM Healthcare Solutions
BHM Healthcare Solutions
http://bhmpc.com/
http://twitter.com/BHMHealthcare
file reviews
newideas@bhmpc.com

"BHM was founded in 2002, and was established to bring together the highest level experts in the healthcare industry. It is the consistent goal of our organization to utilize this expertise to provide valuable guidance and advisory services. BHM has distinguished itself as an industry leader by adhering to the highest professional standards. We believe in leveraging our knowledge assets for the optimal client benefit, and managing client and firm resources in a cost-effective manner. BHM consultants have a unique perspective on the issues which face healthcare, as they have worked in the healthcare payer, hospital, and provider settings at the executive level in positions ranging from AVP to CEO. BHM also differentiates itself by taking a unique data driven approach to all consulting engagements. By basing our analysis and recommendations on fact, rather than opinion, your organization is guaranteed to get measurable and sustainable results. BHM has consistently met or exceeded the expectations of all previous clients, and has done so in a time sensitive and cost efficient manner."

Biologics
Biologics
https://www.biologicsinc.com/
http://twitter.com/BiologicsInc

"Cancer care is complex and often fragmented. So we specialize in cancer care alignment -- empowering payors, biopharma companies, researchers and providers to improve the delivery of services across the cancer care continuum. The Biologics team is driven to make integrative care a reality."

Blue Cross Blue Shield of (insert state here)...
Blue Cross Blue Shield of (insert state here)
multiple sites depending on the state
(some also have variations in their names that don't really include "BC/BS")

Bluegrass Health Network...
Bluegrass Health Network
>   http://www.bhnmanagedcare.com/

"Bluegrass Health Network (BHN) is an innovative provider of medical management services to companies throughout the U.S. BHN has successfully enabled its clients to meet risk management and medical cost containment objectives for Group Health, Workers Compensation, General and Auto Liability and Disability Cases."

Boston Mutual Life Insurance...
Boston Mutual Life Insurance
>   http://www.bostonmutual.com/

"Founded in 1891, Boston Mutual Life Insurance Company has enjoyed a long history of financial strength and stability. Headquartered in Canton, Massachusetts, the company proudly offers a wide range of worksite, group and individual insurance programs nationwide. For more than 120 years Boston Mutual has been a recognized leader in providing flexible insurance products to working Americans and their families through the private and public sectors of the USA."

BPA Health
BPA Health
https://www.bpahealth.com/

"BPA Health connects people to services to improve lives and achieve positive outcomes. On the front lines of our work around the Northwest and nationally, we help people address problems that adversely impact their job performance, health and overall wellbeing. Our established regional roots help us understand and link communities and resources like no large national corporation can. And our deeply held belief that behavioral health is a critical part of overall health motivates our professionals to deliver services with all they have to offer – in mind, body and spirit."

Broadspire
Broadspire
https://www.choosebroadspire.com
http://twitter.com/Broadspire1
customer_relations@choosebroadspire.com

Broadspire provides a full range of claims services including:
Accident and Health
Employer's, Public and Product Liability
General and Product Liability
Marine and Transportation
Property and Business Interruption
Motor (First Party and Third Party)
Personal Injuries
Rehabilitation and Return to Work
Travel, Warranty and Affinity Products
Uninsured Loss Recovery

Brookside Consultants
Brookside Consultants
> https://www.brooksideconsultants.com/
> IME and file reviews

"Brookside Consultants provides nationwide Independent Medical Examinations and related services to its valued clients. Our dedicated experts are here to ensure that you receive high-quality and competitively-priced reports in a timely manner.

In addition to Independent Medical Examinations, we also provide Medical File Reviews, New York State Variance/C4-Authorization Evaluations, No-Fault Examinations, and FCEs."

Bunch and Associates
Bunch and Associates
www.bunchcare.com
http://twitter.com/BunchCare

"Bunch CareSolutions, A Xerox Company, is a national medical management company based in Lakeland, Florida. We operate exclusively in the workers' compensation industry as a full service, managed care firm. Since our founding in 1988, we have consistently grown in size, scope of services and standards of excellence. We have done so without compromising our clinical focus or our mission of "making the world a better place--one life at time."

Using our clinical expertise, we offer innovative and customized managed care solutions focused on quality outcomes and medical cost containment. Because we are passionate and centered on providing programs built on our core competencies--medical case management and medical bill review--we have been highly successful in shortening claim duration, expediting medical recovery and improving financial and return-to-work outcomes for our clients and their injured employees."

C2C Innovative Solutions
C2C Innovative Solutions
www.c2cinc.com
QIC Quality improvement

"C2C Innovative Solutions Inc. (C2C), located in Jacksonville, FL, has proudly served as a Qualified Independent Contractor (QIC) for the Medicare program since the inception of the second-level appeal process in September 2004. Today, C2C is the QIC contractor for several QIC task orders.

C2C fosters an organizational culture that embraces honesty, integrity and respect. We perform our duties with our corporate values in mind: "Integrity, Quality and Value with PRIDE (Passion for our customers, Responsibility to seek innovative solutions, Initiative to make things better, Discipline to strive for excellence and Enthusiasm for the future)."

We have assembled a workforce inspired by a common purpose, of upholding our quality values of "Integrity, Quality & Value driving Continuous Improvement." Our culture generates our drive to deliver exceptional customer service and commitment to upholding the highest quality standards. Our team members have in-depth knowledge of health insurance plans including, but not limited to, traditional fee-for-service (FFS) Medicare, Medicare Advantage (Part C) and Medicare Prescription Drug Coverage (Part D) and vast experience managing second level appeals from case receipt to final disposition."

California Foundation for Medical Care...
California Foundation for Medical Care
    www.cfmcnet.org

"The California Foundation for Medical Care, physician driven, is a unique partnership of twelve Foundations for Medical Care creating one of California's largest and most comprehensive networks dedicated to improving patient access to quality medical care."

California Medical Evaluators
California Medical Evaluators

Cardinal Innovations...
Cardinal Innovations
  https://www.cardinalinnovations.org/
  https://twitter.com/CardinalIHS

"Cardinal Innovations Healthcare is the country's largest specialty health plan, serving 875,000 individuals who are eligible for Medicaid or are uninsured with complex needs throughout North Carolina. Cardinal Innovations pioneered this unique managed care model in North Carolina, which relies on strong community partnerships with providers and stakeholders.

Cardinal Innovations operates at-risk capitated health plans for individuals with complex needs with a commitment to our members that they receive the healthcare services they need to live fuller lives. We maintain a community presence with offices in Charlotte, Chapel Hill, Kannapolis, Concord, Burlington and Henderson."

Care to Care
Care to Care
http://www.caretocare.com/

"Care to Care delivers evidence-based solutions that promote the most efficient and effective use of medical resources across a range of specialties for the benefit of payers, physicians, providers and patients – the right service, at the right time, at the right cost."

CareCentrix
CareCentrix
http://www.carecentrix.com/

"Our teams of highly trained nurses, all experienced in specific disease areas and in managing care to the home, coordinate care with physicians, case managers and network providers. We are URAC accredited for Health Utilization Management (UM) and conduct prospective, and retrospective utilization reviews of requested home care services.* We leverage proprietary data and monitor trends to help enhance the UM policies of our customers, enabling them to make more informed decisions on their coverage policies.

*Our UM decision making is based on the appropriateness of care and services and the existence of benefit coverage. We do not provide financial incentives that promote underutilization and do not reward providers or others for issuing denials of coverage or care."

CareCore National (evicore)...
CareCore National (evicore)
https://www.carecorenational.com/

"Specifically designed with the size and scale to address the complexity of today's and tomorrow's healthcare system, eviCore is a company committed to advancing medical benefits management – and enabling better outcomes for patients, providers, and plans.

Ours is an evidence-based approach that leverages our exceptional capabilities, powerful analytics, and an acute sensitivity to the challenges and needs of everyone involved across the healthcare spectrum. Applying proven talent and leading-edge technology, we harness healthcare's evolving demand and inherent change to realize and deliver improved results for everyone."

Carewise Health http://www.carewisehealth.com/
Carewise Health   http://www.carewisehealth.com/

"Carewise Health offers a series of care management, financial payment integrity, data management, business process management and analytic products and services to health plans, provider health systems, employers and government entities. The combination of technology and key personnel such as nurse clinicians, data and behavioral scientists, actuaries and engineers offer a highly effective partner for customers to achieve their various financial, clinical and operating objectives. Extensive health care and technology domain experience and expertise provides customers with a highly effective solution partner.

Carewise Health, Inc. has been providing Clinical Care Management and Payment Integrity services to employers, unions, health plans, government and providers since 2003. Our focus on data, technology and experienced clinical personnel allows our customers to prove, and improve their care management and payment integrity initiatives."

Careworks
Careworks
http://www.careworks.com/

(multiple companies: CareWorks; CareWorks Absence Management; CareWorks Consultants Inc; CareWorksComp; VocWorks; CareWorks Tech; CWT Interactive)

"One of Ohio's largest managed care organizations, serving over 115,000 employers in Ohio."

"A national leader in FMLA Administration and absence and disability management services."

"Ohio's leading Third Party Administrator for self-insured workers' compensation claims services."

CCME
CCME
http://www.thecarolinascenter.org/
https://twitter.com/MyCCME

"We provide services that help advance the quality and cost effectiveness of health care."

"With over 30 years of quality improvement experience, CCME also provides innovative, cost-effective clinical review services. We assist state Medicaid departments, hospitals, accountable care organizations, and providers of all types manage their data and claims to benefit patients, providers, and payers, simultaneously.

Since 1984, CCME has performed utilization review and quality improvement activities as a CMS-designated Quality Improvement Organization (QIO)--and with the evolution of the system into Quality Innovation Networks--as a Quality Innovation Network-Quality Improvement Organization (QIN-QIO).

CCME is a member of the Atlantic Quality Innovation Network (AQIN), the QIN-QIO for New York, South Carolina, and the District of Columbia, and serves as the QIO for South Carolina."

CE Provider Services...
CE Provider Services
> http://www.ceproviderservices.com/
> Social Security/state disability evals
> info@ceproviderservices.com

"C.E. Provider Services presently performs exams for Social Security and State disability in 9 states and over 45 sites and are continuing to grow. We are also available for insurance physicals, Department of Transportation physicals and other types of exams. Most of our exams take place on Saturdays."

Authors note: If you are interested in performing disability evaluations for Social Security you should discuss your options with the Social Security DDS (disability determination service) near you first. Depending on your situation and the practices in your state you might prefer to simply contract with the state directly instead of a third party organization. See the listing in the directory for Social Security for details.

Cenpatico
Cenpatico
http://www.cenpatico.com/
https://twitter.com/cenpatico

"Since 1994, Cenpatico® has provided comprehensive managed behavioral healthcare services for vulnerable and underserved populations. We started out as a group practice of behavioral health clinicians offering services and care management in Texas. We have never lost our clinical focus and our passion for serving people.

Our members are enrolled in publicly-funded programs including Medicaid (TANF), CHIP, ABD/SSI, the Child Welfare System, and Medicare.

Cenpatico® offers agencies, health plans, and states solutions to administer healthcare services more effectively. Our specialties include managed care solutions for behavioral health, foster care, specialty therapy and rehabilitative services, specialized school services, and community re-entry programs.

We are a national leader in care management. Our programs are tailored to the unique needs of each community we serve. We operate in multiple states with an active local presence. Our members receive care from local teams that truly understand the specific needs of their communities. We continually introduce innovative clinical initiatives and network strategies in all markets, designed to create quality service delivery systems."

Centene
Centene
> http://www.centene.com
> https://twitter.com/Centene

"We are committed to improving the health of the community through health insurance solutions for the under-insured and uninsured, and through specialty services that align with our focus on whole health.

Centene provides health plans through Medicaid, Medicare and the Health Insurance Marketplace and other Health Solutions through our specialty services companies."

CenterPoint Human Services (Cardinal Innovations...

CenterPoint Human Services (Cardinal Innovations Healthcare).

http://www.cphs.org/

"CenterPoint Human Services is now a part of Cardinal Innovations Healthcare.

Individuals in Forsyth, Davie, Stokes and Rockingham counties who receive Medicaid or state-funded services for intellectual or developmental disabilities, mental health or substance use disorders are enrolled in Cardinal Innovations Healthcare's specialty health plan.

Our goal is to make the transition as seamless as possible for members, families and providers. Click on the buttons to the left for additional information. "

Certified Medical Consultants
Certified Medical Consultants
http://www.certifiedmed.com/
IME's

CID Management
CID Management
http://www.cidmcorp.com/
https://twitter.com/CidReview

"The right specialists by your side when you need them.

The Clinical Experience provides all the tools you need to eliminate hurdles and prevent work from coming to a standstill. Whether it's a quick answer to a common question or expert advice on a sensitive topic (or anything in between), we provide the solutions to keep your claims moving forward.

The day-to-day operation of a worker's compensation division is complicated. In fact, it's downright overwhelming. Challenges exist across a diverse group of organizations, from insurance carriers and medical professionals to IT and administrative personnel. Not to mention keeping everything under budget. With so many restrictions, regulations and opinions to deal with, it's inevitable that issues are going to pop up.

And that's why we designed The Clinical Experience.

The Clinical Experience is clinical, regulatory and administrative expertise together with exceptional customer service and superior technology. And best of all, the entire package is available on a claim-by-claim basis. That means no long-term contracts, no red tape and no delays."

Cigna
Cigna
http://www.cigna.com
https://twitter.com/cigna

"Cigna Corporation (NYSE: CI) is a global health service company dedicated to helping people improve their health, well-being and sense of security. All products and services are provided exclusively by or through operating subsidiaries of Cigna Corporation, including Cigna Health and Life Insurance Company, Connecticut General Life Insurance Company, Life Insurance Company of North America, Cigna Life Insurance Company of New York, or their affiliates. Such products and services include an integrated suite of health services, such as medical, dental, behavioral health, pharmacy, vision, supplemental benefits, and other related products including group life, accident and disability insurance. Cigna maintains sales capability in 30 countries and jurisdictions, and has more than 90 million customer relationships throughout the world."

CIME Management
CIME Management
http://www.cimellc.org/
IME
lovinsw@cimellc.org

"The most professional and personal IME Company in the field of medical-expert witness consulting. We concentrate on workers' compensation cases and embrace your IME referrals with a thorough understanding of the meaning of a defense-oriented IME."

CIMRO
CIMRO

http://www.cimro.com/
file reviews
peerreview@cimro.com

"CIMRO is a URAC accredited independent peer review organization serving the public and private healthcare sectors since 1972. Our broad range of services includes quality and utilization management as well as independent peer review / external peer review.

We firmly believe true peer review can only occur when specialties and practice settings between physician and reviewer match. CIMRO's extensive resources include a pool of over 400 clinical peer reviewers in active practice that permits us to attain this goal of effective peer review.

Beyond our commitment to peer-to-peer review, what sets CIMRO apart from our competitors is the fact that at we provide high quality, unbiased peer review at reasonable prices. Our Project Managers assure individualized attention from start to finish to meet the unique needs of our clients."

ClaimsAlliance
ClaimsAlliance
        www.claimsalli.com
        twitter.com/claimsalliance
IME and file reviews

"We provide a comprehensive panel of all specialties throughout the country paired with a myriad of cost containment services for carriers and attorneys. Our entire technology system is built using HIPPA compliant regulatory mandates."

Claims Eval
Claims Eval
www.claimseval.com
http://twitter.com/claimseval1
files reviews claims_eval@claimseval.com

"Claims Eval is a URAC accredited Independent Review Organization providing timely, objective and conclusive reviews to the Workers' Compensation, Disability, Auto, Liability and Group Health markets. Our national peer review panel of credentialed, licensed, board-certified, active practice physicians, are continuously keeping abreast of new developments and standards of care in their fields."

Clinix Healthcare...
Clinix Healthcare
http://www.clinixhealthcare.com/

Utilization Management
Case Management
Disability Management
Disease Management
Medical Claims Review
Independent Review
Health and Wellness Programs
Population Management

CMME of New England
CMME of New England
http://www.cmmeone.com
IME
exams@cmmeone.com

"Central Massachusetts Medical Evaluations was incorporated on 1986 to fulfill a need in the Worcester area for independent medical evaluations. We distinguished ourselves from the beginning as the only Worcester-based company to offer the convenience of a full-service agency. Since then, CMME has grown and expanded to perform evaluations throughout the entire United States. To better reflect our expansion, we became CMME of New England in 1991."

Coastline EAP
Coastline EAP
http://www.coastlineeap.com
EAP

Cognizant
Cognizant
> http://www.cognizant.com
> https://twitter.com/cognizant

"Headquartered in Teaneck, New Jersey (U.S.), Cognizant combines a passion for client satisfaction, technology innovation, deep industry and business process expertise and a global, collaborative workforce that embodies the future of work. With over 50 delivery centers worldwide and approximately 244,300 employees as of June 30, 2016, Cognizant is a member of the NASDAQ-100, the S&P 500, the Forbes Global 2000 and the Fortune 500 and is ranked among the top performing and fastest growing companies in the world."

College Health IPA
College Health IPA
http://www.chipa.com/

"In close partnership with health plans, CHIPA, in alliance with Beacon Health Strategies, helps bring together the fragmented pieces of health care to achieve better results for the people in our care. Our programs are clinically driven, fiscally responsible, and focused on continually improving outcomes for the most complex members.
Since 1991, the College Health IPA (CHIPA) has been providing managed behavioral health services to California residents, making it one of the state's largest regional behavioral health delivery systems to address the issues presented by behavioral health and chronic disease. Beacon Health Strategies is a Massachusetts-based, NCQA-accredited managed behavioral health organization."

Community Health Network of CT...

Community Health Network of CT
http://www.chnct.org/

"Community Health Network of Connecticut, Inc. (CHNCT) is a 501(c) 4 not-for-profit health plan. CHNCT was founded in 1995 by federally qualified health centers who sought to bring non-profit oversight to Medicaid managed care in Connecticut. CHNCT, as a Managed Care Organization for 16 years, served the State of Connecticut's HUSKY and SAGA program populations. Effective January 1, 2012, CHNCT now functions as the state's Administrative Services Organization for the HUSKY Health Program."

Community Health Partners...
Community Health Partners
http://www.chealthpartners.com

"Community Health Partners is a Physician Hospital Organization (PHO) that serves customers in Collier and southern Lee counties. In addition to its network contracting functions, Community Health Partners also offers a variety of other programs."

Community Health Solutions of America...
Community Health Solutions of America
http://www.chsamerica.com/

"CHS is headquartered in St. Petersburg, Florida executing Care Coordination, Population Management and Discharge/Transition of Care services throughout the country. Our team of professionals includes physicians, nurses, social workers and care advocates. CHS, along with its sister organization, Premier Administrative Solutions, a third party administrator, is a multifaceted group experienced in and qualified to manage all aspects of a health care program."

Community Network for Behavioral Healthcare...
Community Network for Behavioral Healthcare
(CommCare) http://www.commcare1.org/

"The Community Network for Behavioral Healthcare, Inc. (CommCare) is a regionally based, provider-sponsored behavioral healthcare firm that offers a variety of managed care products and employee assistance program (EAP) services. Our target market includes private employers, health maintenance organizations, insurance companies, and various governmental agencies."

CommunityCare
CommunityCare
http://www.ccok.com/

"When you choose CommunityCare as your employer, you join a staff of highly motivated individuals who make CommunityCare Oklahoma's best choice for healthcare."

Comp One MCO

Comp One MCO   http://www.componemco.com/

"Our focus is to return the injured worker to the workplace in a safe and timely manner. We provide aggressive case management intervention from the early post injury period. This ensures a complete understanding of all medical concerns surrounding the case. Development of an advocate relationship with the injured worker insures identification of subjective barriers to recovery and allows communication of medical issues to physicians and rehab providers, as well as relating return to work issues to the employer. Open communication with the employer is an essential part of the medical management process. The case manager assists the employer in understanding the employee's injury and rehab needs. These services reduce lost–time and helps our employers with their bottom line costs associated with workers' compensation."

CompManagement Health Systems...
CompManagement Health Systems
    http://www.chsmco.com

"CompManagement Health Systems (CHS), based in Columbus, Ohio, is a workers' compensation managed care organization focused on bringing injured employees back to work safely and quickly.

When a workplace injury causes lost workdays, employer costs escalate, and injured employees need assistance and direction. Our experienced team provides effective managed care services, and designs comprehensive return-to-work programs tailored to meet the needs of our clients and their valuable employees.

With four offices and more than 220 colleagues throughout the state, we know our clients' communities and medical providers."

CompPartners

CompPartners   http://www.comppartners.com/

Medical Provider Networks (MPN) - California Only
Health Care Organizations (HCO) - California Only
Utilization Review Services
Medical and Disability Case Management Services
Physician Peer Review Services
Workers' Compensation PPO Networks
Medical Bill Review Services
First Notice of Injury Reporting Services
A Workers' Compensation Pharmacy PPO Network

Comprehensive Medical Reviews...
Comprehensive Medical Reviews
http://www.comprehensivemedicalreviews.com/
IME/Medical Expert Examinations
Function Capacity Evaluations (FCEs)
Peer Reviews
Radiology Reviews

Concentra
Concentra
http://www.concentra.com
http://twitter.com/ConcentraHealth

"Concentra, a division of Select Medical, is a national health care company focused on improving the health of America's workforce, one patient at a time. Through its affiliated clinicians, the company provides occupational medicine, urgent care, physical therapy, and wellness services from more than 300 medical centers in 40 states. In addition to these medical center locations, Concentra serves employers by providing a broad range of health services and operating more than 140 onsite medical facilities"

Conifer Health Solutions...
Conifer Health Solutions http://coniferhealth.com/
https://twitter.com/coniferhealth

"Conifer Health has been providing managed services to health systems, their health plans and managed populations for more than 30 years. Our value-based solutions enhance consumer engagement, drive clinical alignment, manage risk, and improve financial performance."

Consumers Life (Medical Mutual)...
Consumers Life (Medical Mutual)
http://www.consumerslife.com

"We're an Ohio company, based in Ohio and serving Ohioans with quality life insurance and disability insurance for individuals and employers. Consumers Life is part of Medical Mutual, the oldest and largest health insurance company in Ohio. We're dedicated to serving our community with high quality life and disability products and award-winning service that our members expect."

CoreSource
CoreSource
http://www.coresource.com/

"We provide our clients and their employees with the personal service of a local company, backed by the innovation and resources of a national organization. From each of our local offices around the country, we work every day to provide our clients with comprehensive solutions to their unique employee benefits challenges.

Our focus is administering all aspects of your employee health plan, minimizing its costs and risks, and improving your employees' health and well-being. You control your plan's design and equip your employees with the tools that keep them invested in their own health.

At CoreSource, we know a comprehensive, tightly managed health plan strategy is necessary when it comes to managing medical spend and inflation -- and that's just what our clients receive."

Corporate Care Management...
Corporate Care Management
http://www.corporatecaremgmt.com/

"CCM has over 30 years experience working with self-funded employer benefit plans. Our clients include Third Party Administrators and Self-Administered Employers numbering over 100 benefit plans currently managed. Five of our customers have trusted their members' health and workers' compensation plan benefits to CCM for over 20 years each. CCM has not only demonstrated sustainability in a constantly changing medical and legal environment but, is well known as an innovator so that employer benefits can be as dynamic as the environment in which they must operate.

CCM offers highly customized alternatives to providing case management services. CCM's internally developed IT system integrates all case management functions required for health plan management and total absence management. This assures that cases do not fall through the cracks and strict review time frames are maintained.

CCM provides detailed, informative, and timely periodic reports to demonstrate savings and return on investment at a client level. These reports were specifically created to respond to client's needs and have demonstrated their effectiveness in retaining clients and attracting new business for our TPA clients and foster positive employer-employee relations with our employer clients."

Corporate Health Resources
Corporate Health Resources

http://chr.com/services/independent-medical-evaluations-imes/

CHR is a nationwide examiner network that provides occupational health exams in all 50 states and many international locations as well. Many of our clients have an internal Medical Department and CHR's staff becomes an administrative extension of a company's own department. We coordinate exams outside the catchment area of the company's medical department. For clients without an internal Medical Department, we can provide the same service using your consulting medical director, or physician recommended by CHR.

Corvel
Corvel
http://www.corvel.com/
http://twitter.com/CorvelCorp
IME
"As a national provider of innovative risk management solutions, CorVel helps employers, third party administrators, insurance companies and government agencies control costs and achieve positive outcomes."

Cotiviti
Cotiviti
http://www.cotiviti.com/
https://twitter.com/CotivitiHC

"Cotiviti Healthcare enables payers to achieve accuracy across the payment continuum and improve their financial results with solutions for payer liability, coding and contract compliance, and clinical appropriateness."

Coventry
Coventry
http://www.coventrywcs.com
IME and file reviews

"Coventry Workers' Comp Services offers workers' compensation cost and care management solutions for employers, insurance carriers, and third-party administrators. With roots in both clinical and network services, we leverage more than 30 years of industry experience, knowledge and data analytics. We offer an integrated suite of solutions, powered by technology to enhance network development, clinical integration and operational efficiencies at the client desktop, with a focus on total claims cost."

CPR Risk Management
CPR Risk Management
http://cpr-rm.com/

"Our mission is to combine our knowledge of insurance, risk management and medical best practices in order to assist our clients to evaluate and assess risk from a business and medical perspective."

Cyrca
Cyrca

http://www.cyrcahealth.com/

Managed Carve Out Programs
Marine Medical Management
Excess of Loss
Customized Specialty Medical Programs
Family Planning Programs

D&D Associates
D&D Associates
www.ddassociates.com
IME and file reviews   info@ddassociates.com

D&D Associates provides independent medical
evaluation (IME) and review services, serving the IME
industry since 1984. Our credentialed panel of
physicians and allied professionals conduct physical
evaluations and medical file reviews, delivering
objective, clinically-informed reports to verify the
validity of medical claims.

D&D Associates is accredited by URAC, a leading
healthcare services oversight authority and completes
the SOC 2 audit annually. We have developed an
outstanding reputation for quality services that is due
primarily to the talents and dedication of our team
members.

Dane Street
Dane Street
http://site.danestreet.com
http://twitter.com/danestreet
IME and file reviews

"Dane Street is a national IME and Peer Review organization headquartered in Boston, MA. We are focused exclusively on providing credible, objective and timely examinations and reviews.

We process over 175,000 referrals annually for leading national and regional Workers Compensation, Disability, Auto and Group Health Carriers, Third Party Administrators, Managed Care Organizations, Employers, Pharmacy Benefit Managers and Medicare Set-Aside providers to provide customized IME and Peer Review programs which assist their RNs and Adjusters in reaching the appropriate medical determination as part of the claims management process.

At Dane Street, we are committed to "finishing the job." We realize your referrals to us require careful and timely attention--on each case--from referral initiation to delivery back to your team. Our entire team is committed to consistently meeting your highest expectations around turn-around time, quality, responsiveness, and ease of doing business."

Delmarva Foundation...
Delmarva Foundation
   http://www.delmarvafoundation.org/

"Delmarva Foundation is a national, not-for-profit organization--established in 1973--dedicated to creating solutions to transform health. The company provides leadership services and consultative resources to ensure everyone receives care and services that are safe, effective, efficient, equitable, timely, and person-centered. As a subsidiary of Quality Health Strategies, Delmarva Foundation has long-standing relationships with government agencies and policy-makers as well as other quality improvement stakeholders ensuring quality in these areas:

- Intellectual and developmental disabilities
- External quality review
- Utilization management
- Quality improvement
- Assessing long-term care services
- Improving patient safety
- Reducing health disparities
- Aging

Delmarva Foundation operates offices in Easton and Columbia, Maryland; the District of Columbia; Tampa and Tallahassee, Florida; and Atlanta, Georgia."

Department of Transportation (DOT)
Department of Transportation (DOT)
There are opportunities related to fitness for duty and protecting the public (also see the listing for the FAA).
https://www.transportation.gov/
transjobs@dot.gov

You may also be interested in becoming a "SAP," Substance Use Professional. This is a "person who evaluates employees who have violated a DOT drug and alcohol program regulation and makes recommendations concerning education, treatment, follow-up testing, and aftercare.

As a SAP you represent the major decision point (and in some cases the only decision point) an employer may have in choosing whether or not to place an employee behind the steering wheel of a school bus, in the cockpit of a plane, at the helm of an oil tanker, at the throttle of a train, in the engineer compartment of a subway car, or at the emergency control valves of a natural gas pipeline. Your responsibility to the public is enormous!

As a SAP you are advocate for neither the employer nor the employee. Your function is to protect the public interest in safety by professionally evaluating the employee and recommending appropriate education and/or treatment, follow-up tests, and aftercare." Learn more here: https://www.transportation.gov/odapc/sap

"A Medical Review Officer (MRO) is a person who is a licensed physician and who is responsible for receiving and reviewing laboratory results generated by an employer's drug testing program and evaluating medical explanations for certain drug test results.

As a MRO, you act as an independent and impartial "gatekeeper" and advocate for the accuracy and integrity of the drug testing process. You provide quality assurance review of the drug testing process for the specimens under your purview, determine if there is a legitimate medical explanation for laboratory confirmed positive, adulterated, substituted and invalid drug test results, ensure the timely flow of test result and other information to employers and protect the confidentiality of the drug testing information."
Learn more:
https://www.transportation.gov/odapc/mro

(see also the Drug Testing/ Medical Review Officer listing)

Diamond Medical Examinations...
Diamond Medical Examinations
        http://www.diamondime.com/
IME's
NY and Northeast U.S.
info@diamondime.com

Disability Exam Consultants...
Disability Exam Consultants
http://www.disabilityexamconsultants.com/

Disability RMS
Disability RMS
www.disabilityrms.com

"Disability RMS is the nation's leading provider of turnkey disability risk management products and services. Established in 1993, we offer unparalleled Actuarial, Underwriting and Claims industry expertise in risk management. We offer these services on a reinsured or service only basis."

Drug Testing/ Medical Review Officer
Drug Testing/ Medical Review Officer

There are multiple opportunities for physicians to become a MRO in the workplace drug testing process. This includes interpreting the urinalysis/tox screen and evaluate potential medical explanations for positive results.

If you are interested in this you may wish to start at websites like these (as well as the previous Department of Transportation listing) and subsequently Google "medical review officer"):
https://www.aamro.com/
https://www.acoem.org/MedicalReviewOfficer.aspx

Eastpointe
Eastpointe
http://www.eastpointe.net/

"Eastpointe works together with individuals, families, providers, and communities to achieve valued outcomes in our behavioral healthcare system."

EBMS
EBMS

http://www.ebms.com/
https://twitter.com/EBMS_Inc/

"EBMS is one of the nation's premier industry leaders in health risk management and third party administration of self-funded health benefit plans, designing strategies to transform the health and wellbeing of individuals, organizations and communities."

Eckman/Freeman & Associates...
Eckman/Freeman & Associates
   http://www.eckmanfreeman.com/

"Eckman/Freeman & Associates is an innovative disability management company providing comprehensive medical cost containment for occupational and non-occupational illnesses and injuries. Our customers include workers' compensation, group health, long term disability, and auto/general liability carriers as well as employers and governmental agencies."

EK Health
EK Health
http://www.ekhealth.com/
https://twitter.com/ekhealth

"Providing nurse case management, utilization review/peer review, medical bill review, provider networks, Medicare set aside and other specialty managed care services."

Emblem Health
Emblem Health
http://www.emblemhealth.com/
https://twitter.com/EmblemHealth

Empire State Medical, Scientific and Educational...
**Empire State Medical, Scientific and Educational
Foundation** http://www.esmsef.com/
file reviews

"The Empire State Medical, Scientific and Educational
Foundation, Inc. (Foundation) is a
not-for-profit corporation focused on providing quality
medical review services and DRG/coding validation to
providers and payors at all levels of care. The
Foundation has been involved in medical peer review
activities since 1984 at the State and National levels. We
are URAC accredited as an "Independent Review
Organization: Comprehensive.""

Employers Risk Services (ERS)
Employers Risk Services (ERS) http://www.ers.net/

Episource
Episource
https://www.episource.com/

eQHealth Solutions
eQHealth Solutions
        http://www.eqhs.org/
        https://twitter.com/eQHealth

"Our high-tech and high-touch offerings include innovative medical management systems, face to face community care coordination services, utilization review, clinical data integration and business intelligence analytical reporting – all focusing on increased quality outcomes and optimization of provider and payer networks."

EvaluMed (and EmployMed)
EvaluMed (and EmployMed)
http://www.evalumed.com
IME and file reviews

"EvaluMed®, a privately held Minnesota company established in 1995, is a leading Independent Medical Evaluation (IME) and medicolegal services company. With physician resources that represent over 40 diverse medical specialties, we work to exceed our clients' expectations through superior customer service, innovative product lines, and continuous quality improvement. For medical authority, we are the industry's reliable and credible resource."

Everence
Everence
http://www.everence.com/
https://twitter.com/everence

"Everence is a Christian-based, member-owned comprehensive financial services organization."

eviCore
eviCore

http://evicore.com/
http://twitter.com/evicorehc

"Specifically designed with the size and scale to address the complexity of today's and tomorrow's healthcare system, eviCore is a company committed to advancing medical benefits management – and enabling better outcomes for patients, providers, and plans.

Ours is an evidence-based approach that leverages our exceptional capabilities, powerful analytics, and an acute sensitivity to the challenges and needs of everyone involved across the healthcare spectrum. Applying proven talent and leading-edge technology, we harness healthcare's evolving demand and inherent change to realize and deliver improved results for everyone."

Eviti
Eviti

http://www.eviti.com/

"eviti is an innovative, collaborative approach to improving access to the most appropriate, evidence-based treatment for each individual patient, and facilitating more efficient communication between oncologists and insurers in any cancer care setting. Through eviti's end-to-end oncology decision support platform, oncologists access, at the point of treatment prescribing, unbiased and actionable information regarding the latest evidence-based treatment regimens.

eviti also provides an online forum, including peer-to-peer review and validation of treatment plans, for resolving treatment plan decision disparities. The result: everyone wins. Physicians receive access to the most up-to-date evidence-based protocols along with the assurance of expedited payment from participating payer organizations. Insurers receive transparency of risk and assurance that they are paying for quality treatment, and patients receive the peace of mind they are receiving the best possible evidence-based care."

EVOnational
EVOnational
http://www.evonational.com
IME

"Welcome to EVOnational, a revolutionary advancement in the claims industry. EVOnational is a personalized shared network bridging the gap between claims professionals, physicians, and claimants creating a partnership to ensure a seamless claims management process. We provide the resources allowing you to actively monitor, service, and expedite your claim process with an EVOnational "partner" by your side at all times. Our superior service and state of the art technology have superseded the industry standards and have created an invaluable partnership for managing claims. Through precision, efficiency, and dramatic cost savings to you EVOnational has become a revolutionary resource to claims professionals worldwide."

Exam Coordinators Network
Exam Coordinators Network
http://www.ecnime.com/

"ECN (Exam Coordinators Network) provides a wide array of services to assist clients in managing the cost of medical claims and cases. We procure and provide the highest quality independent medical examinations, medical record and radiology reviews, FCE's, Return-to-Work, and Fitness for Duty examinations, FMLA and ADA reviews from our nationwide network of experienced medical experts in all medical specialties and allied health professions.

Our clients include but are not limited to: insurance carriers, third party administrators, attorneys, human resource professionals, public and private disability insurers, nurse case managers, risk managers, retirement funds, hospital risk managers, and other entities who need our medical evaluation services."

ExamNet (Texas)
ExamNet (Texas)
http://www.theexamnet.com/
emailexamnet@gmail.com

ExamWorks
ExamWorks
http://www.examworks.com/
IME and file reviews   info@examworks.com

———

"ExamWorks Group, Inc. is a leading provider of independent medical examinations, peer reviews, bill reviews, Medicare compliance, case management, record retrieval, document management and related services.

We provide IME services through our medical panel of credentialed physicians and allied medical professionals. Our independent medical review process is fully contained within our private cloud network. Custom portals, applications, workflow enhancements and systems integration are part and parcel of our service, all included for the price of an IME service.

Our clients include property and casualty insurance carriers, law firms, third-party claim administrators and government agencies that use independent services to confirm the veracity of claims by sick or injured individuals under automotive, disability, liability and workers' compensation insurance coverages.

We help our clients in the U.S., Canada, the United Kingdom and Australia manage costs and enhance their risk management processes by verifying the validity of claims, identifying fraud and providing fast, efficient and quality IME services."

Experience Claims Management (NY)...
Experience Claims Management (NY)
 http://experienceclaims.com/
IME and file reviews

Experts.com

Experts.com
http://www.Experts.com
https://twitter.com/experts_com
experts directory/advertising

Express Exams, inc.
Express Exams, inc.
http://expressexams.com
IME

"AT EXPRESS EXAMS, INC., we strive to be the most
professional company in the field of liability cases and
embrace your IME referrals with a thorough
understanding of your case. We recognize that all
companies have different approaches to similar
challenges. Our product is the service we provide. Most
Law Firms and Adjusters simply do not have the
resources or time to spend researching or credentialing
proper experts and scheduling IME's. With your
demanding workloads, why not let our team facilitate
this for you. We have years of experience in the IME
and expert witness fields. Try us on your next case."

ezURs
ezURs
http://www.ezurs.com

Services include Utilization Management, Case
Management, Bill Review, Peer Review, Independent
Medical Evaluations, Pharmacy Review

Federal Aviation Administration (FAA) Fitness for...

Federal Aviation Administration (FAA) Fitness for Duty Evaluations on pilots

If you have questions you may wish to contact a regional flight surgeon:
http://www.faa.gov/licenses_certificates/medical_certification/rfs/

A good contact for psychologists is Chris Front, Psy.D.:
Chris.Front@FAA.gov
More information:
https://www.faa.gov/other_visit/aviation_industry/designees_delegations/designee_types/ame/ametraining/prospective_guide/

Federal Hearing and Appeals Services
Federal Hearings and Appeals Services, Inc.
117 West Main Street
Plymouth, PA 18651

Toll Free: 800-664-7177
PH: 570-779-5122
FX: 570-719-0306
http://fhas.com   @FHAS_inc

1. Who can providers contact to discuss working with your organization (and how should they contact them)?

Medical professionals interested in becoming members of FHAS's medical review panel can contact Laura Desciak, HR Manager/Credentialing Specialist, at LDesciak@fhas.com or 570-779-5122 x1462.

2. Which types of health care providers do you recruit? For example, do you recruit only physicians or do you also recruit psychologists, chiropractors and other disciplines.

Currently, we are recruiting all medical professionals, including Psychologists, Clinical Social Workers, Dieticians, Physical Therapists, Occupational Therapists, Physicians, Doctors of Medicine (M.D.), Doctors of Osteopathy (D.O.), Doctors of Dental Surgery (D.D.S.), Doctors of Medical Dentistry (D.M.D.), Doctors of Podiatric Medicine (D.P.M.), Doctors of Optometry (O.D.), and Doctors of Chiropractic/Chiropractors (D.C.). The physicians must be American Board certified and represent all medical specialties and sub-specialties recognized by the American Board of Medical Specialists and American Dental Association.

3. What types of services do you tend to offer in relation to medical records reviews and/or IME's?

FHAS provides internal and external medical review and peer review services for multiple federal and state programs.

4. Do your opportunities require the professional to be in active clinical practice and if so how is active clinical practice defined (ex: number of hours per week/ percentage of income from direct treatment)?

Medical Practitioners performing internal reviews must have at least five (5) years of full-time equivalent experience providing direct clinical care to patients, have a scope of licensure or certification and professional experience that typically manages the medical condition, procedures, treatment or issue under review, and if an M.D. or D.O. must have a Board certification by a medical specialty board approved by the American Board of Medical Specialties or the American Osteopathic Association. If a D.P.M., must have a Board certification by the American Board of Podiatric Surgery or the American Board of Podiatric Orthopedics and Primary Podiatric Medicine.

Medical Practitioners performing external reviews must have all of the requirements for internal reviews but also must have provided direct clinical care to patients within the past three (3) years.

5. What opportunities, if any, do you have for professionals who are not currently in active clinical practice?

FHAS employs medical professionals who are not actively practicing to perform internal medical reviews.

6. Are you recruiting providers on a nationwide level or are there particular areas of the country you work in (if so which areas of the country are you currently recruiting in)?

FHAS is current recruiting medical professionals on a national level, as we perform internal and external medical review services throughout the country.

7. Do you have a description of your company and what you do that you'd like to have included in the company directory of the book?

Established in 1996, FHAS is certified with the U.S. Department of Veterans Affairs (VA), Center for Verification and Evaluation (CVE), as a Veteran-Owned Small Business (VOSB). FHAS has also been verified by the Commonwealth of Pennsylvania as a Small, Diverse Business (SDB), and Veteran Business Enterprise (VBE). In addition, FHAS holds full URAC (Utilization Review Accreditation Commission) accreditation as an Independent Review Organization (IRO) for both internal and external comprehensive reviews.

As one of the leading providers of medical claims' review services, analysis, and adjudication services, FHAS has processed over 1.5 million reviews and written reports on behalf of government agencies since its foundation. In the past year alone, FHAS's staff completed approximately 200,000 case reviews, in which all cases were properly processed, scheduled, and adjudicated with a 100% timeliness rate of completion.

In order to successfully issue quality medical reviews, FHAS utilizes a network of Board-certified physicians and other healthcare professionals with diverse specialties, who have the appropriate education, experience, and expertise to render decisions for internal and external review requests.

8. If possible (and it is understandable if you can't), can you estimate what you typically pay to consultants or otherwise describe as much about how consultants are paid as possible?

Medical consultants are hired as independent contractors and are reimbursed on a per-case basis. We would rather not provide rates as they are often contract specific and vary.

First Choice Evaluations...
First Choice Evaluations
www.firstchoiceevaluations.com
IME and file reviews

"The industry leader Worldwide in providing Independent Medical Evaluations for Workers Compensation claims, No-Fault claims as well as Liability cases to insurance companies, third party administrators, self-insured companies, and law firms. We have a large database of physicians Worldwide to meet all of your IME needs.

First Choice Evaluations prides itself with its reputation of integrity and its experienced professional staff. We offer the highest quality service with quick turnaround times and competitive pricing.

First Choice Evaluations offers to our clients the following enhanced services: prompt appointments, fast delivery of written reports along with file copying. All examinations and peer review services are performed by skilled BOARD CERTIFIED PHYSICIANS."

First Choice Health Network
First Choice Health Network
http://www.fchn.com

"First Choice Health (FCH) is a Seattle-based, physician and hospital owned healthcare company. We have provided network, administrative and clinical services to the Northwest since 1985. We now serve well over one million people with our array of products and services in Washington, Oregon, Alaska, Idaho and Montana through our network affiliate Health InfoNet.

First Choice Health PPO (FCH PPO) is a large multi-state PPO (Preferred Provider Organization) that includes hospitals, facilities, and professional providers who have agreed to discount their fees to members of FCH PPO. First Choice Health Administrators (FCHA) offers employers transparent administrative solutions combining the latest in technological sophistication, health plan controls and leading edge analytics. First Choice Health Medical Management (FCH MM) provides cost saving strategies for our clients and members as well as management services that optimize a members' health status, well being, productivity and access to quality healthcare. First Choice Health Assistance Services (FCH EAP) offers tailored strategies and services to support organizations such as; businesses, associations, trusts and physician groups."

First MCO
First MCO
http://www.firstmco.com/

"First MCO is a full-service managed care organization providing medical cost containment services for workers' compensation programs, auto insurers, and group health. With more than 30 years in the industry, we help insurance companies, insurance funds, third-party administrators, and self-insured employers manage their costs, associated with workers' compensation and other medical claims. Among other things, we offer URAC accredited Case Management, Network Access, Negotiation and Bill Review services. Our medical claims management process is built on and reinforced by the guiding principles of patient welfare, sustainable quality, and active collaboration with our clients and customers."

Focus Health
Focus Health
http://www.focushm.com/
Independent Review Organization
File review

Freelance Physician...
Freelance Physician
https://freelancephysician.com/
(mainly temp staffing)

Future Care http://www.futurecareinc.com/
Future Care http://www.futurecareinc.com/
IME

"Future Care is a provider of national and international medical care management services. The company assists medical claims payers in adapting cost containment and medical care management solutions to the environment mandated by the U.S. Federal Jones Act, the International Seafarer's Law, Workers Compensation and International Healthcare."

Gallagher Bassett
Gallagher Bassett
> www.gallagherbassett.com
> https://twitter.com/gbtpa

"With a cornerstone on Claims Management, we've grown. Now we bring the same, premier service that's become the GB hallmark to an array of services. Each with unrivaled strength and expertise. Discover how we can help with:

Claims Management
Risk Control Services
Technology & Analytics

With more to come, so watch this space. GB isn't simply embracing the changes in insurance and risk management. We're creating them. Defining the opportunities and setting the standard for others to follow."

Genex
Genex
http://www.genexservices.com
http://twitter.com/gbtpa

IME and file reviews

"Genex is the most experienced managed care provider in the industry, delivering clinical services and solutions that improve productivity, contain costs, and help injured workers get better faster. As managed care specialists, workers' compensation payers and risk managers rely on us to achieve superior results through expertise, assured quality, and responsive program design. We address the unique needs of each company and each injured employee, building trust one relationship at a time."

Employment: hr@genexservices.com
Referrals
referral@genexservices.com
Social Security
genexdisability@genexservices.com
Provider Panel Requests
panelrequests@genexservices.com
Provider Nominations
provider.nominations@genexservices.com

GenRe
GenRe
http://www.genre.com/
http://twitter.com/Gen_Re

"Gen Re delivers reinsurance solutions to the Life/Health and Property/Casualty insurance industries."

Greeley
Greeley
http://greeley.com/

"The Greeley Company has an outstanding reputation for providing solutions through consulting, education, interim staffing, credentialing management, and external peer review to healthcare organizations nationwide. We focus on contemporary needs and challenges related to medical staff optimization & physician alignment; accreditation, regulatory compliance & quality; and credentialing & privileging."

Group Benefit Services (GBS)
Group Benefit Services (GBS)
http://www.g-b-s.com/

"Group Benefit Services, Inc. (GBS) is the premier employee benefit plan administrator in the Mid-Atlantic region. Since 1980, GBS has continued to develop creative solutions that help employers achieve their business goals. Our efficient administration, advanced technology, cost containment strategies and creative benefit designs allow our clients to realize their strategic benefit plan and financial objectives."

GSG Associates
GSG Associates
http://www.gsga.net

"Founded in 1994, by Registered Nurses, GSG Associates, Inc. provides unique cost-containment solutions through specific programs designed to meet our client's needs in the Workers' Compensation, Employee Management and Disability Management industry.

GSG has focused our services on the experience of our founder and Management team, who have over 70 years experience in providing Medical and Disability Management services in a variety of venues and industries.

GSG differentiates ourselves from our competitors in the approach we take to our services: GSG has always brought an Advocacy approach to our work for our clients. GSG believes that if we ensure the injured, or ill, employee receives the appropriate care at the appropriate time from the appropriate provider, and receives the appropriate work restrictions, the employee will experience the best outcome and the employer will be assured that waste is eliminated from the equation. We simply want to do the right thing for injured workers, and employers."

Guardian Life Insurance
Guardian Life Insurance
www.guardianlife.com
http://twitter.com/guardianlife

"As a mutual insurance company, we are owned by our policyholders who share in Guardian's actual financial results through annual dividends. These payments are determined by the firm's profits, and Guardian has paid a dividend every year since 1868. We take the very long view, invest soundly, and maintain a strong capital base that enables us to meet our insurance commitments today and far into the future. Our sole responsibility is to our clients and policyholders, and that is reflected in everything we do."

H.H.C. Group
H.H.C. Group
http://www.hhcgroup.com/
file reviews

"Our staff of licensed health Insurance adjusters who are attorneys, nurses, pharmacists, physicians, and other health insurance professionals, will contact providers to negotiate/reprice your costly medical claims. Patients can submit/enter claims directly online for pricing reductions. Providers can use this site to electronically submit claims to health insurers."

Health Advantage...
Health Advantage
http://www.healthadvantage-hmo.com/
      http://twitter.com/arkbluecross

"Health Advantage is the state's largest and oldest health maintenance organization (HMO), serving over 225,000 members in every county in Arkansas."
Health Alliance Plan

Health Alliance Plan
Health Alliance Plan
www.hap.org
http://twitter.com/hapmichigan

Health Care Excel
Health Care Excel
http://www.hce.org/

"Health Care Excel (HCE) is a healthcare technology company focused on helping clients improve their quality ratings and optimize their revenues. Our combination of leading-edge data services and clinical expertise has positioned us as a strategic partner in the transformational change of the quality and integrity of healthcare systems.

Our team includes highly skilled data analysts, technology experts, clinicians and coders from the medical, dental and behavioral health sectors to ensure measurable results through a variety of services including Star Ratings, Pay-for-Performance, commercial risk adjustment, and more."

Health Care Service Corporation...
Health Care Service Corporation
        http://www.hcsc.com/

Health Care Service Corporation (HCSC) is the largest customer-owned health insurance company in the United States. HCSC offers a wide variety of health and life insurance products and related services, through its operating divisions and subsidiaries; including Blue Cross and Blue Shield of Illinois , Blue Cross and Blue Shield of Montana , Blue Cross and Blue Shield of New Mexico , Blue Cross and Blue Shield of Oklahoma , and Blue Cross and Blue Shield of Texas The company employs more than 22,000 people and serves more than 15 million members.

Health Claim Solutions...
Health Claim Solutions
      http://www.healthclaim.net/
file reviews

HealthClaim Solutions® provides full service Medical Review for Healthcare Organizations, Disability Administrators, Pharmacy Benefit Managers, Dental Benefit Plans. Considine & Associates is a URAC-accredited Independent Review Organization.

HealthClaim Solutions® also provides claims and coding review for outpatient surgery to address coding abuse for in- or out-of-network providers.

HealthClaim Solutions® offers a national panel of over 450 specialist physicians and other health professionals from 125 specialties to provide file review.

Health Design Plus
Health Design Plus

http://www.hdplus.com/

Fully integrated health care services including PPO network management, medical management and claims administration.
Comprehensive utilization management, medical case management and patient advocacy, the core businesses of Health Design Plus:
Precertification of patient admissions, outpatient services and specialized services
Case management and discharge planning
Discount negotiations
Concurrent and retrospective medical claims review
Individualized PPO network development and management, fostering provider relationships that produce maximum access for employees and cost savings for clients:
Network of providers balancing access and cost
Contract negotiations
Websites and directories listing hospitals, physicians and ancillary providers
Ongoing network management
Assigned Customer Service Representatives focused on caller needs, problem solution and customer satisfaction.
Access to Good Health by Design suite of services:
Wellness Counts®, LifeStyle Management
Lifestart®, Maternity Management
CareWise®, Demand Management
HealthLiving™, Disease Management Programs
Monthly/Quarterly and Annual Reviews to provide data and analysis for making decisions about the health care Plan.

Regular meetings with the Health Design Plus Team to set goals, review service utilization and claims, identify trends and determine course of action.

Health Information Designs...
Health Information Designs
> http://www.hidesigns.com/
> https://twitter.com/thePAexperts

"Our range of services are designed to fill the clinical gaps in your organization. With solutions built on decades of experience in clinical service, customer support, workflow processes, pharmacy benefit management, and quality assurance, we provide value that stabilizes your foundation and improves member care."

Health Integrated...
Health Integrated
> http://www.healthintegrated.com/
> https://twitter.com/hintegrated

"Health Integrated enables health plans to effectively manage their members and control costs through Precision Empowered Care Management."

Health Management Partners
Health Management Partners
> https://www.hmpsd.com/

"Health Management Partners is an independent provider of innovative health management programs that are tailored to individuals and customized to companies. We offer solutions to organizations that help bring healthcare costs under control while improving quality care in the healthcare system.

Health Management Partners has been serving clients for over 15 years. As a proven leader in medical management services, our team of professionals provide solutions to employers, health plans and members.

Our services include:
Wellness
Health Screenings
Conditions Management
Case Management
Utilization Management
Preauthorization"

Health Management Solutions (HMS)...
Health Management Solutions (HMS)
> http://www.hmssolutions.com
> http://twitter.com/HMSMco

"HMS is an Ohio MCO certified to medically manage workers' compensation claims in Ohio. Our goal is to return injured employees to work quickly and safely. HMS is a provider owned MCO with access to the resources of an integrated healthcare system. Employers have a single point of contact and access to a team of professionals led by an experienced nurse case manager."

Health Net Federal Services
Health Net Federal Services
https://www.hnfs.com/

"For 25 years, Health Net Federal Services, LLC (HNFS) has partnered with the Department of Defense to provide health care to service men and women and their family members. Through the TRICARE® program, HNFS assists approximately 2.8 million beneficiaries including active duty, retired, National Guard and Reserve, and family members. Health Net Federal Services was one of the first companies in the U.S. to develop comprehensive managed care programs for military families.

In addition, HNFS partners with Department of Veterans Affairs (VA) to provide high quality health care and community support.

MHN Government Services provides behavioral health programs and serves millions of active duty service members, and National Guard and Reserve members, and provides family member services related to deployment and reintegration.

Health Net Federal Services' mission is to help people be healthy, secure and comfortable."

HealthCare Partners
HealthCare Partners
http://www.hcpnv.com/
      https://twitter.com/HCP_nevada

"HealthCare Partners Medical Group is a network of more than 310 primary care physicians and more than 1,700 specialists. With medical clinics and specialty care affiliates throughout Pahrump, Las Vegas, North Las Vegas, Henderson, Mesquite and Boulder City, HealthCare Partners Nevada (HCPNV) is committed to delivering the highest quality to care to all of our patients.

Through our total care model, HealthCare Partners provides patient centered comprehensive primary care, specialty care, urgent care and hospice services. Founded in 1996, HealthCare Partners Nevada is an affiliate of HealthCare Partners LLC with offices in California, Florida and Nevada."

Healthcare Resources NW...
Healthcare Resources NW
      http://healthcareresourcesnw.com/

"Organized in 1995, Healthcare Resources NW (HRNW) is a nonprofit organization that consists of a broad system of healthcare professionals and providers who have developed an integrated approach to contracting relationships and the effective delivery of best-practice healthcare services.

HRNW is dedicated to providing a seamless path of care, which is quality driven and cost effective. We believe this approach generates greater continuity of care and satisfaction among our patients and our physicians, as well as a more value-added collaborative relationship with our payors.

Functions & Capabilities include:

Network, contracting and management
Case Management
Claims Management and Processing
Credentialing"

HealthCare Strategies
HealthCare Strategies
http://www.hcare.net/

"During our 30 years in business, HCS has earned a reputation for delivering quality services as a medical management provider and now through technology platforms by offering next generation, informatics-driven, health management services used singularly, or in tandem, with our highly effective clinical programs.

HCS deploys its sophisticated technology platform, deep domain experience, and skilled clinical staff to merge predictive analytics, risk stratification and evidence based interventions into effective programs that will improve outcomes and reduce overall healthcare costs. These unique capabilities allow HCS to accurately predict high cost medical care events, proactively manage patient health, provide highly effective interventions, as well as positive clinical and financial outcomes."

HealthHelp
HealthHelp
http://www.healthhelp.com/
https://twitter.com/HealthHelp

"HealthHelp collaborates with payors and providers to ensure patients receive the right care at the right place and at the right time.

Our educational and consultative process has improved long-term outcomes and
reduced costs for the healthcare industry."

HealthSmart
HealthSmart
http://www.healthsmart.com/
https://twitter.com/HealthSmartCare

"Whether you're an employer, member, provider, payor or broker, HealthSmart has a solution for you. We offer a wide array of healthcare options and can create a unique solution for your organization. Our flexible, customizable healthcare plans meet the needs of our clients.

Who Uses HealthSmart and Why?
Employers look to HealthSmart to find cost effective, comprehensive healthcare coverage without the restrictions of a fully insured plan. Our self-funded insurance plans give employers more control over plan design, help manage costs and increase cash flow, as well as offering administrative and technical support to help meet healthcare objectives.
HealthSmart members have access to numerous services on our website, designed to help improve the quality of their health and control healthcare costs. Members can visit our Wellness Resource Center for health-related information, use our Provider Search to find a physician or local hospital and register through eServices to manage their account information. Providers use HealthSmart services because they benefit from our established provider networks that offer a stable patient base and expedited claims turnaround time. When you become a HealthSmart provider, we provide a range of seamless services to help you with your business.

Payors rely on our expertise in the areas of cost containment, provider network management, utilization review, precertification and other management services. Our services facilitate clean claims, resulting in reduced administrative costs and improved customer service.

Brokers who partner with us can take advantage of our innovative scope of services, national presence and competitive plans.

HealthSmart is dedicated to providing superior products and services to all of our customers, clients, consultants and brokers. We'll find a custom solution to meet your specific needs!"

Healthways
Healthways
http://www.healthways.com/
http://twitter.com/Healthways

"At Healthways, our business is improving well-being. Understanding needs within customer populations. Engaging individuals in sustained behavior change that helps them live longer, happier, more productive lives.

Healthways has always been at the forefront of healthcare transformation. More than 30 years ago, we started with programs to support diabetes care, progressed to help set the first national standards for disease management, evolved to support the continuum of health across populations, and finally expanded our scope from physical health to overall well-being improvement.

Why? We embrace the World Health Organization's definition of health as "a state of complete physical, mental and social well-being and not merely the absence of disease or infirmity." Healthier people cost less and perform better, which is the value proposition we offer our clients."

Helmsman TPA (Liberty Mutual)
Helmsman TPA (Liberty Mutual)
  www.helmsmantpa.com
  https://twitter.com/HelmsmanTPA

"Helmsman Management Services is a third party administrator that offers claims management, managed care, and risk control solutions for businesses with complex risk management needs."

Highmark
Highmark
www.highmark.com
http://twitter.com/highmark

"Highmark Inc. is a national, diversified health care partner serving members through its businesses in health insurance, dental insurance, vision care and reinsurance. Our mission is to make high-quality health care readily available, easily understandable and truly affordable in the communities we serve."

Hines & Associates
Hines & Associates
www.hinesassoc.com

"Hines & Associates is a nationwide
and independent leader in personalized managed
healthcare, focusing on what is important to you--
comprehensive services with the program excellence
and cost containment that you demand."

HMS
HMS
http://hms.com/
http://twitter.com/hmshealthcare

"Today we are the most comprehensive cost
containment company for healthcare payers in
America. Using innovative technology as well as
powerful data services and analytics, our solutions
cover the entire payment continuum:

Eligibility verification
Payment accuracy
Fraud identification and prevention
Cost savings
Performance improvement
Provider education

Based in Irving, Texas, HMS has more than 2,300 employees in 25-plus offices across the country. We are a wholly owned subsidiary of HMS Holdings Corp., traded on NASDAQ (ticker: HMSY), and certified by HITRUST. HMS is URAC-accredited for Health Utilization Management: Vendor Certification. Permedion, a wholly owned subsidiary of HMS, is a QIO-like entity, and is URAC-accredited for Independent Review Organization: External Review and Health Utilization Management. With the support of our leadership, we also promote social responsibility."

Hoover
Hoover
http://www.hooverinc.com/

"With nearly 40 years of experience managing workers' compensation for commercial carriers, employers and government, Hoover has the medical and insurance expertise, leading-edge technology, human and business resources, and organizational flexibility to help our customers rise above workers' compensation challenges. Our strength is in our service, and we offer a level of stability and continuity rarely found in the workers' compensation marketplace. Our customers' satisfaction is our core value, and is behind every service we provide.

As business needs change in the new economy, we will continue to expand and refine our services, streamline processes and workflows, and embrace new technologies - all in support of our commitment to helping our customers manage the impact and control the costs of workplace injury and illness."

HQSI
HQSI
http://hqsi.org/
http://twitter.com/HQSICorp
file reviews

"Since its founding, HQSI has designed, implemented, and evaluated hundreds of successful quality improvement projects, and reviewed more than three million medical records for a diverse client base.
For more than three decades, HQSI partnered with the Centers for Medicare and Medicaid Services (CMS) as New Jersey's Quality Improvement Organization (QIO). We continue to partner with CMS as part of a regional Quality Innovation Network-Quality Improvement Organization (QIN-QIO).
Using our evidence-based, data-driven approach, we have also partnered with governmental (state), private, for profit and not-for-profit organizations to make healthcare safer, more accessible and more cost-effective."

Human Behavior Institute...
Human Behavior Institute
http://www.hbinetwork.com/

"Founded in 1990, Human Behavior Institute (HBI) is a full-service behavioral health organization headquartered in Las Vegas, Nevada. As a leader in the development of effective quality assurance programs, HBI is devoted to excellence in clinical care and customer service, and adheres to URAC and NCQA standard of quality.

HBI develops and implements managed behavioral health services and employee assistance programs. Unlike others, HBI is the only behavioral health managed care company that has specialty clinics allowing members the flexibility of choosing a network provider and the option to attend supportive services through HBI's staff model.

HBI's approach to behavioral health care is innovative, dynamic, solution-focused, and diverse – where the clinical practice is interdependent with managed care obtaining data from these two integral functions in order to develop and implement targeted programming to address issues and provide solutions. Accountability, creativity, and measurable outcomes are hallmarks of our behavioral care products."

Humana Behavioral Health...
Humana Behavioral Health
   www.humanabehavioralhealth.com

"What makes Humana Behavioral Health a smart choice? We are committed to changing health behaviors to improve lives. For more than 20 years, our commitment to well-being has resulted in positive outcomes for employers, health plans and insurers. Our approach integrates the care of the mind and body – treating both the physical and mental together - to enhance health, and to increase personal and workplace productivity. Humana Behavioral Health proudly serves more than 5 million members and offers extensive health behavior resources."

Humana Military
Humana Military
      https://www.humanamilitary.com/

"Humana Government Business, Inc. is a wholly owned subsidiary of Fortune 100 health and wellness company Humana Inc., headquartered in Louisville, Ky.

Humana Government Business combines the full spectrum of Humana's capabilities with our unique, government-focused operations and experience. Humana is one of the nation's largest publicly traded health benefits companies and a leader in consumer engagement, providing guidance that leads to lower costs and a better health plan experience throughout its diversified customer portfolio.

A TRICARE Managed Care Support Contractor since 1995, Humana Government Business partners with the Department of Defense as Humana Military to provide healthcare services to approximately 3 million active duty and retired military and their families in the South Region of the U.S. The company supports 53 Military Treatment Facilities in the states of Arkansas, Alabama, Florida, Georgia, Kentucky, Louisiana, Mississippi, Oklahoma, South Carolina, Tennessee and Texas."

IEC Group
IEC Group
www.iecgroup.com
http://twitter.com/IECGroupHR

"Firmly established as an experienced and trusted partner, organizations of all sizes have utilized our numerous consulting services for more than 50 years. Assessing an organization's needs and implementing effective solutions is our top priority. We have a team of consultants with vast experience and a variety of advanced degrees who have strategically designed tools and services to ensure results.

As organizations strive to remain competitive, outsourcing non-core business competency has developed into a powerful trend. AmeriBen · IEC Group is an expert in providing key human resource services for growing, stable, and downsizing organizations. From bundled to custom-tailored services, AmeriBen · IEC Group can develop a program that meets the needs of the organization as well as the defined budget."

IMCS group
IMCS group
https://www.theimcsgroup.com/

"INTEGRATED MEDICAL CASE SOLUTIONS (IMCS)
The IMCS Group is a national network of clinicians
utilizing an evidence-based biopsychosocial functional
model of disability.

Our assessments and interventions assists claimants to
overcome return to work barriers, return to function
and settle cases.

This benefits the claimant and their family, the
employer, the carrier and society as a whole.

IMCS Clinicians are experts in Workers' Compensation
and Disability Evaluation and provide:

COPE with Pain Psychologists for Chronic Pain
Management
COPE with Trauma Psychologists for Employees
exposed to Trauma events
Functional Medicine Evaluations (FME)
Functional Psychological Evaluations (FPE)
Mental Heath Disorders Fit For Duty Screening
Opioid Fit For Duty Screening"

iMedReviews
iMedReviews
http://www.imedreviews.com/
info@imedreviews.com

"We Specialize in providing independent medical peer reviews by helping physicians, insurance companies, hospitals, HMOs, and state departments of insurance control healthcare costs, and do what's right for each patient, every time."

"Our independent medical peer reviewers can aid in answering questions including but not limited to:
Medical Necessity
Experimental/Investigational
Standard of Care
Pre Authorizations
Hospital Admissions
Length Of Stay
Level of Care
Billing and Coding
Disability
Workman's Compensation"

IMX Medical Management Services...
IMX Medical Management Services
   http://www.imxmed.com
   IME and file reviews
   discoverimx@imxmed.com

"IMX Medical Management Services is a national medical consulting company, which specializes in Independent Medical Evaluations, Functional Capacity Evaluations, Medical Record Reviews and Occupational Health Services. We recruit, credential, coordinate, schedule and deliver quality reports on these medical services throughout the United States. IMX Medical Management Services recruits only highly qualified Board-Certified Physicians for Medical Evaluations and Medical Record Reviews, and Physical and Occupational Therapists for Functional Capacity Evaluations.

PRODUCTS & SERVICES
Independent Medical Evaluation
Second Medical Opinions
Defense Medical Evaluations
Functional Capacity Evaluations
Peer or Medical Record Reviews
Occupational Medical Consultative Services
Ergonomic Assessments
Job Analyses"

Independent Claim Consultants Network (ICCN)
Independent Claim Consultants Network (ICCN)
http://www.independentclaims.net
IME and file reviews

"Independent Medical Evaluations:

Procurement of IME providers involves a lengthy and meticulous process designed to assure that the quality of the IME interview and report is exceptional and reliable. We diligently utilize measures to make certain that IME experts are qualified by degree and certification, and that they are sophisticated, unbiased, critical thinkers who are adept at addressing the specific and often complex issues characteristic of these cases.

IME reports can be murky and incomplete, or they can be clear, well-founded in data, and thorough. In order to obtain a comprehensive report of an in-depth evaluation, ICCN's IME provider search begins with a review of work samples and continues with detailed interviews with potential expert applicants. The process of pursuing a forensic evaluation must include a discussion with potential providers to confer about the complex assessment process and to ensure that each evaluator has the experience and skills to provide outstanding work.

Medical File and Peer Reviews

ICCN offers unparalleled file and peer review services nationally and internationally, relying on a network of specialists of the highest caliber. With access to experts in the psychiatric and medical fields, ICCN assists in effectively assessing and managing complex psychiatric and co-morbid claims in the disability, worker's compensation, property/casualty, wrongful death, and personal injury arenas.

Medical record reviews are conducted by experts chosen for their expertise in the condition(s) relevant to each specific case. These reviews are comprehensive and clearly address your questions. ICCN has developed pointed and concise questions for our reviewers. Our process, however, is designed to utilize or to incorporate your questions, as well. Our staff will work with you to develop the most productive questions for each review.

Peer reviews should enhance the claims process in numerous and potentially pivotal ways. When it is possible to conduct a professional collegial interview, our Peer Reviewers engage the treating doctor in meaningful discourse about the claimant's clinical status and functional capacity. This intervention, when done well, sheds a bright light on the case and establishes the opportunity for a productive resolution to otherwise intractable cases. Our summary reports include details of a thorough interview, with data to support conclusions. Treating doctors are provided with a copy of the interview and a request for their signature to assure that the report is accurate.

ICCN's peer reviewers perform exemplary work, assisting the referring claims examiner or case manager in synthesizing and interpreting data as part of early intervention, on-going cases, or in long-standing cases that have seen little progress."

Independent Evaluation Services, inc.
Independent Evaluation Services, inc.
http://www.ies-ime.com

opportunities@ies-ime.com

"We are an IME vendor that is actively growing our national network to better accommodate our client needs"

<u>Independent Medical Evaluation Company...</u>
Independent Medical Evaluation Company
> http://www.imecnys.com/
> referral@imecnys.com
> NY State IME's

"Independent Medical Evaluation Company (IMEC), LLC, provides expert, independent medical opinions about your injury or medical condition that are clear, concise, and credible.

IMEC's panel of board certified physicians conducts the independent medical evaluations and presents an independent opinion to the legal profession, insurance carriers, third party administrators, and other entities. IMEC is an independent medical evaluation company, and we comply with state, federal, and national regulations. We normally have medical evaluation reports processed in three days. This is unheard of in our industry, and it is a very big point of pride for us. We coordinate everything involved, from scheduling and performing the evaluation to reviewing the reports for accuracy."

<u>Independent Medical Evaluations, PC...</u>
Independent Medical Evaluations, PC
> https://www.imei.com/

IME and file reviews

"Independent Medical Evaluations, PC has been the forefront of providing medical legal services since 1986. With over 18,000 screened and board-certified Specialty Providers, we have one of the largest National databases available. Our medically educated team coordinates the entire process to provide you with punctual and professional independent analysis and documentation for your case. We strive to provide individualized services to accommodate your company's needs."

Independent Medical Expert Consulting Services...
Independent Medical Expert Consulting Services (IMEDECS)
http://www.imedecs.com
file reviews

"IMEDECS is a national independent review organization known throughout the healthcare industry for its high-quality medical reviews, extensive panel of experts, and responsiveness to client and regulatory needs. Some of the clients who benefit from IMEDECS' services include, but are not limited to, hospitals, managed care organizations, third-party administrators, employer groups and state agencies throughout the United States.

What We Specialize In

. Case Reviews

. Quality/Hospital Peer
. Med. Cov. Policy Evals
. Disability Reviews
. Coding Reviews/ DRG Validation/ Claims Analysis
. Dispute Resolution Services
. Government Services"

Independent Physical Exam Referrals (IPER)...
Independent Physical Exam Referrals (IPER)
> http://iperinc.com/
IME and file reviews
iperinc@aol.com

"IPER was established to provide the insurance industry with a cost-effective and efficient method of scheduling independent medical examinations and peer reviews."

Industrial Medicine Associates (the IMA group)
Industrial Medicine Associates (the IMA group)
http://www.industrialmed.com/
http://twitter.com/TheIMAGroup
http://twitter.com/IMArecruiting
contact@ima-us.com

"Headquartered in Tarrytown, New York, with its main operations center in Albany, New York, The IMA Group is a national leader with a reputation for providing high-quality medical, psychological and speech and language evaluations. We focus on Social Security Disability, Employability, and Independent Medical Evaluations, and Occupational Health Services. Our clients include local, state, and federal agencies, as well as private insurers and corporations."

Authors note: If you are interested in performing disability evaluations for Social Security you should also discuss your options with the Social Security DDS (disability determination service) near you. Depending on your situation and the practices in your state you might prefer to simply contract with the state directly instead of a third-party organization. See the listing in the directory for Social Security for details.

Inetico
Inetico
http://www.inetico.com/

"Provides healthcare cost containment services to self-funded, fully insured and travel plan members across the United States and Puerto Rico."

Innovative Care Management...
Innovative Care Management
http://www.innovativecare.com/

"Innovative Care Management has over 20 years of experience in providing the highest quality service in the Medical Management community. Ranked "Best in Class" by an international consulting firm, we are a URAC accredited healthcare management company specializing in working with self-insured employers, Taft Hartley trusts, and various Tribal entities. Our current client base is nationwide and our technology easily allows us to partner with TPAs throughout the United States."

"Preauthorization & Utilization Management
Case Management
Healthy Mother Baby
Disease Management
Medical Director Services
Controlled Substance Monitoring Program
24×7 Nurse line
Telehealth 24 x 7 Doctor Line"

Integra
Integra
http://www.integrahealth.com/

"Whether you need efficient, accurate plan administration, focused and compassionate medical management, or the convenience of an onsite clinic, we offer a comprehensive program tailored to an employer's unique set of goals. Spanning the entire continuum of healthcare, our services are fully integrated and competitively priced, resulting in higher quality care and a smarter utilization of every group benefit dollar.

Founded in 1983 as Benefit Management Services, Inc. (BMS), today Integra Employer Health, a Maestro Health company, is a leading independent group benefits administrator and member health services company. Based in Charlotte, North Carolina, Integra Employer Health, a Maestro Health company, currently provides superior service to plan members throughout the United States and across diverse range of industries."

Integrated Medical Evaluations
Integrated Medical Evaluations
http://www.imewest.com/physicians/

Integrated Medical Referrals...
Integrated Medical Referrals
> http://www.integratedexams.com/
> IME
hr@integratedexams.com

"Integrated Medical Referrals, Inc. (IMR, Inc.), provides comprehensive administrative and technical support to physicians and allied health professionals, such as chiropractors and psychologists, conducting medico-legal services for the insurance and IME industry. We have been in the industry for more than a decade and have established an excellent reputation for our integrity and ethical practices. We possess a solid infrastructure, which includes both knowledgeable personnel and the latest cutting edge computer technology allowing us to serve physicians and the IME industry at the highest possible level. We provide only 'non-medical' administrative and support services. We do NOT make any medical determinations nor do we provide any medical treatment."

" • Independent Medical Examinations in No-Fault, Workers Compensation, Disability and
    Liability cases conducted in one of our examining offices or in a physician's treating office.
• Independent Medical Examinations can also be conducted at a patient's home or in a nursing
    home, if necessary.
• Peer reviews including Bill Reviews and Variance Reviews (for Workers Compensation
    cases).
• Hospital File Reviews.
• Disability Reviews.
• Causality Reviews.
• Insurability Reviews.
• Expert Witness Testimony, including court testimony and depositions."

Integrated Risk Services
Integrated Risk Services
http://integrated-risk.com/
NY WORKERS' COMPENSATION INDEPENDENT
MEDICAL EVALUATIONS

Integrity
Integrity
http://integrityme.com
Integrity Medicolegal Enterprises
4800 Olson Memorial Highway
Suite 250
Minneapolis, MN 55422
Phone: 763.398.5300
Toll-Free: 1.877.528.1757
Fax: 763.398.0491

Internationational Healthcare Consultants, inc.
Internationational Healthcare Consultants, inc.
http://www.ihcatl.com/

"Over the years, IHC has expanded its focus and
enviable reputation to now include all areas of medical
expertise. We provide a specialized analysis of medical
cases in virtually all medical specialty areas. Support of
these medical consultations is provided by engineering
and other scientific evaluations as they are relevant to
each particular claim issue. In addition, we can arrange
onsite special investigations where this tool is helpful
in evaluating the case.

At all times, IHC requires that its consultants maintain total objectivity in each and every file. Our reports provide comprehensive reviews of the information provided, with an emphasis on the fairness of the determination and conclusions which are presented. IHC offers its objective evaluations to attorneys and any other professionals who may have need of objective scientific and medical forensic reporting."

International Medical Group
International Medical Group
> www.imglobal.com
> https://twitter.com/imglobal
> hr@imglobal.com

"For more than 25 years, IMG has dedicated its efforts to providing international medical insurance, travel insurance and impeccable service to the international community. It's our specialty. We realize that traveling abroad can be an exciting experience. We also know that anything can happen while you're away from home - whether visiting short-term or living abroad indefinitely. It's important to be prepared for any unexpected illness, injury or medical emergency. Many traditional medical plans simply are not designed for international travel.

IMG's combination of insurance products and unparalleled services bring Global Peace of Mind®. We've served millions of people worldwide in more than 170 countries. Our products supply the coverage you need, while our services help overcome language, currency, time zone and cultural challenges."

# # #
IPRO
IPRO
http://ipro.org/
https://twitter.com/IPROorg
file reviews

"IPRO works to improve the quality and value of healthcare services by:

Partnering with Providers to Improve Care/Health Outcomes

IPRO works to improve patient care by partnering with healthcare providers across all settings, including hospitals, nursing homes, hospice programs, dialysis centers, physician practices and more.

Ensuring Medically Necessary and Appropriate Care

IPRO evaluates patient care from perspectives of medical necessity, quality of care, appropriateness of decision making and length of hospital stay, as a safeguard against unnecessary and inappropriate medical care.

Promoting Value-Driven Healthcare

IPRO supports government agencies and other stakeholders in developing health information technologies, data sharing, and incentive programs that facilitate cost and quality transparency and promote evidence-based best practices."

# # #
ISG
ISG
http://isgvalue.com/
IME and file reviews

"ISG is a national market leader and industry pioneer delivering a unique suite of medical and anti-fraud related insurance management services to employers, third party administrators, insurance claim markets, the disability industry and group health administrators."

# # #
J.P. Farley
J.P. Farley
http://www.jpfarley.com/
http://twitter.com/jpfarleycorp

"J.P. Farley Corporation founded in 1979 by Jim Farley, current President and CEO, is a privately-held third-party administration and consultation firm. The company was founded to deliver added value to employee benefit Plans that are self-funded for medical, prescription, dental, vision, short-term and long-term disability benefits. Flexible Spending Accounts (FSA), Health Reimbursement Accounts (HRA), and Health Savings Accounts (HSA) administration are also part of the portfolio of service offerings.

J.P. Farley Corporation inaugurated care management services to provide additional managed care plan features prevalent in the industry. Our team demonstrates the importance of providing the highest quality care management for our customers in everything that they do from personal, caring patient interactions to the plan savings reported back to our clients."

JBAmedical
JBAmedical
https://www.jbamedical.us/

# # #
JEC Disability Management...
JEC Disability Management
        http://jecdisabilitymanagement.com
IME; case management
jecdisability@aol.com

"JEC Disability Management
is a private company devoted to the goal of providing complete and efficient medical cost containment and related services for the injured and disabled.

JEC Disability Management
services insurance companies, self insured companies, third party administrators, unions and attorneys.

We recognize that all companies have different approaches to similar challenges. It is our philosophy that our product is the service we provide. At JEC Disability Management, we make the utmost effort to meet each individual client's specific needs in order to assist in the goal of reducing claims costs.

The current principals ofJEC Disability Management are Carole Bronfman RN CCM and Emily Fernandez. Ms. Bronfman is a registered nurse trained in critical care and is a certified Case Manager. Ms. Emily Fernandez has been the director of IME Services for the past 12 years in charge of credentialing panel physicians. The principals have been in the IME/Peer/Film Review and Medical Case Management business for the past 16 years. As a result, JEC has been voted the preferred vendor by major insurance companies examiners."

# # #
Juris Solutions
Juris Solutions   http://www.jurissolutions.com
IME, expert witness

# # #
Jurispro
Jurispro
http://www.jurispro.com/
expert witness

# # #
KePRO
KePRO
http://www.kepro.com
file reviews

"Since 1985, KEPRO has helped more than 20 million members lead healthier lives through clinical expertise, integrity and compassion. KEPRO was founded by physicians and clinical expertise is at the core of our organization.

We are a leading quality improvement and care management organization. We offer innovative and outcomes-focused solutions to reduce the unnecessary use of health care resources and optimize the quality of care for public and commercial clients. KEPRO's tailored programs maximize members' quality of life, and realize greater cost savings for members and clients alike.

KEPRO is on a journey to transform medical management and to develop customized solutions tailored to our client's specific business requirements, while improving the quality of life for patients, reducing costs, and achieving return on investments for our clients. Our approach to medical management is holistic and compassionate and is coordinated around a patient's entire healthcare experience.

KEPRO's comprehensive, member-centric care management solutions go far beyond traditional utilization and case management by coordinating the care provided to members with acute, chronic and complex conditions.

Headquartered in Pennsylvania, KEPRO also has offices in California, Florida, Illinois, Maine, Maryland, Massachusetts, Minnesota, Ohio, Oklahoma, Oregon, South Carolina, Tennessee, Virginia, Wisconsin and West Virginia. KEPRO is URAC accredited in case management, health utilization management, and disease management. We are also National Institute of Standards and Technology (NIST) and Federal Information Security Management Act (FISMA) certified.

Our goal is to build healthier communities in partnership with our clients. Our values are promises we keep every day. And why we keep growing with our clients."

# # #

Landmark Healthcare http://www.lmhealthcare.com/
Landmark Healthcare
    http://www.lmhealthcare.com/

"Landmark's mission is to assist health plans in the delivery and management of their physical medicine benefits, more specifically physical, occupational and speech therapy, chiropractic, spine surgery and interventional pain procedures. Our goal is the efficient delivery of superior clinical outcomes through the dissemination and adoption of evidence-based medicine. Our management programs rely on data analytics; we profile the practice patterns of providers to identify those whose resource utilization deviates materially from their peers on a risk-adjusted basis. We work with these providers to encourage patient-centered treatment regimens that focus on functional restoration.

We recognize that our management is only as good as the clinical foundation of our expertise and so we concentrate our resources on the development and maintenance of our clinical practice guidelines. Moreover, we employ experienced clinicians to interpret them in a manner that reflects the real world challenges faced by practitioners every day. Finally, we believe that transparency and frequent communication with providers strengthen working relationships, which in turn lead to better clinical outcomes.

We are a highly focused organization. Landmark serves the health plan market exclusively and only in the realm of physical medicine. Our executive team is comprised of former health plan executives and clinicians who understand the complexity of group health insurance, from both a systems and regulatory perspective. Finally, we know that a health plan's success is determined by its relationships with its employer groups and members, who are heavily influenced by their experiences with individual providers. Our goal is to help those providers achieve success because their success is ultimately ours.

Landmark was founded in Los Angeles in 1985. We now serve seven million health plan members across the country. Landmark is based in Sacramento, California with satellite offices in four other states."

# # #
Liberty Mutual
Liberty Mutual
>   www.libertymutual.com
>   https://twitter.com/LibertyMutual

"Liberty Mutual Insurance helps people preserve and protect what they earn, build, own, and cherish. Keeping this promise means we are there when our customers need us most.

Throughout our operations around the world, we are committed to providing insurance products and services to meet the needs of individuals, families, and businesses; offering a diverse and dynamic work environment for our employees; and supporting our communities."

# # #
Lincoln Financial
Lincoln Financial
www.lfg.com
http://twitter.com/lincolnfingroup

"Lincoln Financial Group provides advice and solutions that help empower Americans to take charge of their financial lives with confidence and optimism. Today, more than 17 million customers trust our retirement, insurance and wealth protection expertise to help address their lifestyle, savings and income goals, as well as to guard against long-term care expenses. Headquartered in Radnor, Pennsylvania, Lincoln Financial Group is the marketing name for Lincoln National Corporation (NYSE:LNC) and its affiliates. The company had $223 billion in assets under management as of June 30, 2016."

# # #
Linkia
Linkia
http://www.linkia.com/

"Linkia is a specialty healthcare company dedicated solely to Orthotic & Prosthetic (O&P) management and care. Linkia offers simplified network management and administration, in-depth industry expertise, and scalability to meet the unique needs of your organization."

# # #
Logical IME
Logical IME
http://logicalime.com/

# # #
Logistics Health (LHI)
Logistics Health (LHI)
www.logisticshealth.com
VA disability evals

"We deliver care through a nationwide network of medical, dental and behavioral health providers.

Our network is comprised of a wide variety of specialties to help us meet the diverse needs of our customers. Through our network we're able to coordinate physical exams, dental exams and treatment, immunizations, periodic health assessments, vision and audio services, drug and alcohol testing and several other diagnostic and screening services."

LHI is a subsidiary of OptumHealth Holdings, Inc., part of the UnitedHealth Group (UHG) family of businesses.

# # #
Lumetra Healthcare Solutions...
Lumetra Healthcare Solutions
      http://lumetrasolutions.com/
file reviews

"Lumetra Healthcare Solutions Health Information Technology Support Services: A customizable suite of services that will help you optimize HIT, increase efficiencies, maximize incentive payments and improve patient care."

"As a URAC-accredited Independent Review Organization (IRO) and a designated QIO-like entity, Lumetra maintains a diverse range of clients on the local, national, and international level. Our affiliation with IPRO, a New York based, national healthcare assessment and improvement organization, strengthens our service offerings to our clients."

# # #
Madison National Life
Madison National Life   www.madisonlife.com

"MNL was founded in 1961, and is headquartered in Madison Wisconsin. The Company is licensed in 49 states, American Samoa, the District of Columbia, Guam, and the Virgin Islands, and is an authorized reinsurer in the State of New York. Madison National Life is rated A-(Excellent), for financial strength, by A.M. Best, a widely recognized rating agency that rates insurance companies on their relative financial strength and ability to meet their obligation to their insureds (An A++ rating from A.M. Best is its highest rating).

Madison National Life is involved in several lines of life, health and disability business including:

Group Term Life, Short-Term Disability and Long-Term Disability for both public and private sector employers across the country."

# # #
Magellan Health
Magellan Health
http://www.magellanhealth.com/
http://twitter.com/MagellanHealth

We move beyond the traditional by delivering behavioral health and employee assistance program services; specialty health, including musculoskeletal, cardiac, advanced imaging management and physical medicine; and integrated care management to health plans, employers, Medicaid, Medicare and the Federal government.

# # #

Magellan Rx Management
Magellan Rx Management
http://magellanrx.com
http://twitter.com/Magellan_Rx

"At Magellan Rx Management, we are a full-service pharmacy benefits manager (PBM) that specializes in solving complex pharmacy challenges for our customers. We believe in developing and executing smart solutions that leverage our industry-leading experience and technology to exceed expectations across the following lines of business:

Employer, Third Party Administrator, Broker
Managed Care
Government, Medicaid, Medicare Part D
As a pioneer in medical specialty pharmacy management and a leader in best-in-class formulary optimization programs, we deliver consistent, proven cost savings. As clinical experts, we deliver customized programs to address our clients' most pressing clinical challenges, drive STAR improvements, and engage patients and providers to deliver improved health outcomes.

Welcome to a unique vision of care.

Magellan Rx Management is a division of Magellan Health, Inc."

# # #
MagnaCare
MagnaCare

http://www.magnacare.com/
http://twitter.com/magnacare

"For nearly 20 years we've kept New York and New Jersey healthy with our unrivaled MagnaCare Network, giving you access to the best healthcare pros around. Regardless of your industry or unique healthcare needs, we have the best solution for you - keeping quality at its peak and costs way down."

# # #
ManageAbility IME
ManageAbility IME
http://www.manageabilityime.com/
Info@manageabilityime.com

# # #
Martin's Point
Martin's Point
http://martinspoint.org

"Martin's Point is a health care organization leading the way to provide better care at lower costs in the communities we serve. As a not-for-profit organization, our primary mission is helping our patients and health plan members live healthier lives, treating each one with warmth, care, and concern. Our administrative offices are located in Portland, Maine, though our health plans and Health Care Centers have a much broader reach in Maine and beyond."

# # #
Mass Mutual
Mass Mutual

www.massmutual.com
http://twitter.com/massmutual

"MassMutual is a leading mutual life insurance company that that is run for the benefit of its members and participating policyowners. MassMutual offers a wide range of financial products and services, including life insurance, disability income insurance, long term care insurance, annuities, retirement plans and other employee benefits."

# # #
Maximus
Maximus
http://www.maximus.com/
http://twitter.com/MAXIMUS_news

file reviews; ex: Medicare appeals

"Since 1975, MAXIMUS has operated under its founding mission of Helping Government Serve the People ®, enabling citizens around the globe to successfully engage with their governments at all levels and across a variety of health and human services programs. MAXIMUS delivers innovative business process management and technology solutions that contribute to improved outcomes for citizens and higher levels of productivity, accuracy, accountability and efficiency of government-sponsored programs. With more than 16,000 employees worldwide, MAXIMUS is a proud partner to government agencies in the United States, Australia, Canada, New Zealand, Saudi Arabia and the United Kingdom."

"MAXIMUS is the national leader in providing government health plan enrollees and providers with independent appeal decisions of health insurance denials. Since 1989, the Centers for Medicare and Medicaid Services (CMS) have relied upon us for conflict-free resolution of Medicare appeals.

Today we receive more than 600,000 appeals claims a year for Medicare Parts A, C, and D. We also serve the U.S. Office of Personnel Management Federal Employees Health Benefits Plan (FEHBP), and more than 48 state health insurance regulatory agencies.

The MAXIMUS Federal team of health appeals professionals includes subject matter experts in quality of care, independent review and human subject protection. We employ full-time medical directors, health attorneys, pharmacist-attorneys, nurse-attorneys, nurse professionals and podiatrist-attorneys. Our fully credentialed national panel of more than 500 physicians and other reviewers represent every recognized medical specialty and all major licensed practitioner categories."

"Our national movement towards managed care frequently pits the needs of patients against health plan budgets. Patients have the right to appeal adverse decisions through independent external review organizations like MAXIMUS.

MAXIMUS is the sole external review organization for Medicare Parts A, C, and D. As a Qualified Independent Contractor (QIC) for CMS, we serve as the administrative vendor for the entire QIC program (AdQIC).

We also provide professional and timely medical reviews for the US Office of Personnel Management, which oversees health plans for employees of the US Federal government, as well as for more than 30 state regulatory agencies.

Join our National Panel of Health Care Reviewers

MAXIMUS offers a wide range of opportunities for qualified physicians and other practitioners, such as chiropractors, podiatrists, speech pathologists, physical and occupational therapists, and other health professionals. A qualified applicant may work as an off-site independent consultant or as an on-site hourly employee in one of our offices. Many of our consultants find case review to be intellectually rewarding and a welcome added dimension to their clinical activities.

Qualifications

If you are a health care professional and would like to join our national panel of reviewers, you must:

Be a graduate of an accredited school
Hold an active and unrestricted license in your state of practice

Be board certified by an ABMS or AOA recognized
board
Hold a valid DEA certification, if applicable
Have a minimum of 5 years active practice experience
Have malpractice insurance coverage, if actively
practicing
Have no history of disciplinary actions
Be in active practice a minimum of 24 hours a week as
required for some projects but not required for all on-
site work"

# # #
McKesson
McKesson
http://www.mckesson.com/
http://twitter.com/mckesson

"McKesson is the oldest and largest health care
company in the nation, serving more than 50% of U.S.
hospitals, 20% of physicians and 96% of the top 25
health plans. We deliver one-third of all medications
used daily in North America."

# # #
MCM
MCM
http://www.medicalcost.com/
http://twitter.com/MCM_MEDCOSTMGMT

"A pioneer in medical management, Medical Cost Management Corporation, dba MCM Solutions for Better Health, was founded by Michael O'Connor in 1986 to meet the population health management needs of self-funded plans, Taft-Hartley Trusts, associations, and claim payers. MCM is a physician directed company that is URAC accredited and licensed in all states with requirements. They are a leading provider of population health management programs that cover the entire continuum of care. MCM and its subsidiary Med-Care provide services to over 550 plans representing over 600,000 members on a nationwide basis."

# # #
MCMC
MCMC
http://www.mcmcllc.com
http://twitter.com/mcmcllc
IME and file reviews
info@mcmcllc.com

"MCMC offers a full suite of managed care services to the Workers' Compensation, Group Health, Auto-No Fault and Disability markets. In addition, MCMC also offers managed care services to other entities including the ERISA, FELA, FMLA, General Liability, Longshore and Texas Nonsubscriber markets.

Our services reduce medical costs while our innovative technology solutions like Zebra® increase efficiencies for clients. We continually exceed the expectations of our clients through exceptional customer service and ongoing quality initiatives. In addition, we offer flexibility and ease of use which has led us to become a recognized industry leader in providing managed care services.

Unlike other managed care service companies, MCMC offers clients a flexible service model which allows program customization including sourcing or leasing options, and bundling or unbundling of services. This model provides clients a strategic alternative to match their individual operating structure.

MCMC has a premier management team consisting of several key executives with well over 300 years of collective managed care service experience. MCMC's management team's goal is to provide a new service and processing solution geared towards customized client specific offerings for partnering and sourcing of services."

# # #
Med Control Evaluation...
Med Control Evaluation
> http://www.medcontrolny.com/
> IME and file reviews

"We are an Independent Medical Evaluation company that has been providing nationwide IMEs, Peer Reviews and Record Reviews for the past 22 years. All the doctors in our panels are Board certified in their specialties. We ensure that all New York State Workers' Compensation Board mandates are strictly adhered to, and all HIPAA rules and regulations are followed. Med Control Evaluation provides IME's for Workers' Compensation, No-Fault and Liability claims for insurance companies, third-party administrators, law firms and self-insured.

We credentialize all doctors and they are available to testify. All appointments get confirmed with the Claimant and/or Attorney and Doctor two days before the IME is to take place, so as to minimize no-shows. The narrative report is received within five days and reviewed to make sure that all needed information is included. All IME requests get answered within 24 hours of receipt and communication with all parties is initiated.

Appointment Services:
-Physicians located within claimant's community
-Exams scheduled within 24 hours of receipt of assignment
-More than 1,800 board certified physicians throughout the United States
-Wide choice of specialties, including gastroenterology, neurology and orthopedic surgery
-All physicians are available for testimony at hearings or depositions
-Quality control checks: every report is reviewed by a claims professional"

# # #

MedCom Care Management...
MedCom Care Management
> http://www.medcomcaremanagement.com/

"Our Population Health Management program provides your organization with a combination of proactive education and personal solutions. Both are key features - and they work in tandem to create a fully integrated approach. Each feature specifically pinpoints the appropriate level of care for each individual. Our strategic outreach plan addresses the entire healthcare continuum, improving all risk categories: acute, chronic, diagnosed, and healthy/at risk. And the personal outcome - and related cost savings - speak for themselves. Gilsbar's Population Health Management program is guided by full-time Medical Directors and over forty Clinicians and Registered Nurses serving our members in every state.

Utilization Management
Case Management
Chronic Care Management
Maternity Management
Wellness
Oncology Management
Transplant Care Management
Behavioral Health
Advocacy Services
Data Analytics and Validation"

# # #

MedCost
MedCost
http://www.medcost.com/

"MedCost LLC is an integrated benefits solutions company offering customized programs to help employers lower their health plan costs and provide more affordable benefits for their employees. We are based in Winston-Salem, North Carolina, and work with employers and health care providers throughout North Carolina, South Carolina, and Virginia to bring them smart solutions that get real results. They rely on our strategic benefit plan design, flexibility in benefit administration, best-in-class care management programs, and customer-focused service.

At MedCost, we regard our clients as partners, and our constant goal is to establish a standard of exceptional service and provide smart, comprehensive health plan solutions that are flexible, customer-focused, customized, and integrated. Our family of products and services are designed to yield real results by helping manage costs and encouraging health and wellness for employers in the Carolinas, Virginia, and beyond:

Care Management – innovative, customized employee care management programs including utilization management, transitional care management, catastrophic case management, maternity management, nurse health coaching, telehealth services, gaps in preventive care, and many more health and wellness programs.

Benefit Solutions – full-service, integrated third party administration through MedCost Benefit Services, offering a broad range of products and services, including medical and dental administration, stop loss, and flexible spending account and COBRA administration.

Networks – a vast network of MedCost providers throughout the Carolinas, including all hospitals and over 45,000 physicians. And, for MedCost Benefit Services' clients outside the Carolinas, an exclusive partnership with Virginia Health Network to offer MedCost Ultra in Virginia, along with relationships with national networks for primary network and travel.

MedCost was founded in 1983 and is jointly owned by Carolinas HealthCare System and Wake Forest Baptist Health. MedCost Benefit Services was formed in 1998."

# # #
Medecision
Medecision
http://www.medecision.com
http://twitter.com/MEDecision

"Healthcare organizations partner with us to successfully take on calculated clinical and financial risk"

# # #
Med-Eval
Med-Eval

http://www.med-eval.com/

"Med-Eval is a leading provider of independent medical evaluations and discounted medical diagnostic testing for the workers' compensation, automobile, general liability, and non-occupational disability claims industries."

# # #

Medex Analytic Services...

Medex Analytic Services

http://www.medexservice.com

IME and file reviews   info@medexservice.com

"Medex Analytic Services is the preeminent provider of Independent Medical Examinations, Peer Reviews, Radiology Reviews, and Medicare Set Asides for medical and legal comprehensive analysis of automotive, bodily injury, workers compensation, and liability claims. Our nationwide service assists our clients in managing and analyzing their medical claims.

Our clients consist of insurance carriers, self-insured entities, municipalities, attorneys, third-party administrators and more. Our partners can expect the highest level of medical expertise, responsiveness, quality, and professionalism structured within the strict compliance requirements of the regulatory environment in which they operate.

Medex provides elite services with a management team that possesses over 70 years of experience in all areas of medical management and claim administration. Our board certified panel of physicians represent the leaders within their vast specialties. The panel is constantly monitored to ensure that our team of physicians maintain the highest level of expertise and integrity. Medex is dedicated to providing a level of service and knowledge that exceeds industry expectations and standards. We are client oriented, accurate in quality assurance, and provide our clients with industry changing technology. Medex's core goal is to develop a partnership with our clients which allows us to become a resource of knowledge. We will accomplish this by committing to a policy of ongoing training and continual education."

# # #
Media Referral
Media Referral
http://mediareferral.com/
IME and file reviews

"Media Referral Inc. is a full service vendor company which schedules and coordinates independent medical examinations, radiology reviews and peer reviews regarding liability, workers' compensation and no-fault claims on behalf of insurance companies, self insured companies, third-party administrators and defense attorneys."

# # #
Medical Audit & Review Solutions...

Medical Audit & Review Solutions
> http://www.marsauditor.com/
> info@marsauditor.com

# # #
Medical Consultants Network (MCN)...
Medical Consultants Network (MCN)
> http://www.mcn.com/
IME and file reviews

"What We Do

Independent Medical Examinations
Medical Peer Reviews
Bill Review Services
Utilization Reviews
Areas of Expertise

Short and Long-Term Disability
Workers' Compensation
Auto/PIP/Casualty/Liability
Independent Review Organization (IRO) Services"

They were kind enough to respond to the survey:

·   Is there a good contact person/department to give to physicians and/or psychologists in relation to recruitment/credentialing with your organization? Is there a desired contact method (ex: an email address or phone number) for them?

206.219.4941; 800.636.3926; RECRUITING@mcn.com

·   Do you contract directly with psychologists and/or neuropsychologists for medical records file review work or IME's?   Yes

·   Do you work directly with psychologists and/or physicians or do you go through third party companies? If so, which companies do you tend to use? Generally we work with them directly and do not usually go through third party companies.

·   Do you contract directly w/ physicians for medical records file review work or IME's?   Yes.

·   Do you ever have any employment opportunities for psychologists and/or neuropsychologists? No, the IME and Peer review work is all done on a contract, per case basis only.

·   Do you ever have any employment opportunities for physicians? No, the IME and Peer review work is all done on a contract, per case basis only.

·   If you employ psychologists and/or physicians, do you allow them to work from home? n/a

·   Do you ever have any employment or contract opportunities for nurses in relation to file reviews and/or IME work? Yes, MCN has nurses in our Client Services/Report Review Department.

·   Do you ever have any employment or contract opportunities for mental health counselors/social workers in relation to file reviews and/or IME work? No.

·   Do any of your opportunities require the professional to be in active clinical practice and if so how do you define active clinical practice? (ex: how many hours per week? What percentage of income from direct treatment?)

·   What opportunities, if any, do you have for professionals who are not currently in active clinical practice?   It is not required in most cases but it is frequently preferred and is tracked; active practice is defined as 8 hours per week or more, with some individual client definitions as well.

·   Do you contract/employ professionals nationwide or are there particular areas or regions of the country you work in; which areas of the country are you currently recruiting in?   We contract and are recruiting for all regions nationwide.

·   Which physician specialties are you actively recruiting right now? Orthopedic Surgery, Psychiatry, PM & R, Neurology, Occupational Medicine, Neurosurgery.

·   Are you actively seeking psychologists or neuropsychologists right now?   Yes

·   Can you provide estimates of a typical fee range that you tend to pay to psychologists and/or physicians for medical records file review and IME work (ex: do you have a typical hourly fee or per case fee/ per report fee that you are able to share)? Psychologists tend to be paid less than physicians. Per file review, $200 is a standard price. Per IME, a flat rate of $400 - $500 is standard. Many doctors do charge hourly rates of $250/hour as well. These are estimates, however, and price is often dictated by location and experience.

·   Can you provide a brief company description that you'd like included in the book? Medical Consultants Network (MCN) was founded in 1985 in Seattle, WA. Originally a regional company, MCN created the first national network of independent medical providers in 1997, and we now serve all fifty states and Canada. We understand that as a physician (or any type of medical professional), you could choose to work for any number of service providers. Our network of providers (24,000 options and growing) choose to work with MCN because we put medical expertise and medical integrity at the heart of everything we do.

# # #

Medical Equation http://medicalequation.com/
Medical Equation   http://medicalequation.com/

"Since 1996, our panel of fully licensed, board certified physicians and professional staff have delivered objective, evidence-based medical record reviews in a swift and professional manner. Medical Equation, Inc. (MEI) provides a wide range of utilization review services to meet the emerging needs of the workers' compensation community."

# # #
Medical Evaluators...
Medical Evaluators
        http://www.medicalevaluators.com
IME (Ohio) and file reviews

# # #
Medical Expense Management...
Medical Expense Management
        http://www.medexpense.com/
IME and file reviews   referrals@medexpense.com

"Providers of Independent Medical Evaluations to insurance companies, self-insured employers, and TPA's for Workers' Compensation, Auto No-Fault, and Liability claims in All States."

# # #
Medical Management Group of New York...
Medical Management Group of New York
        http://www.medicalmanagementime.com
        IME and file reviews
info@mailmmg.com

"Since 1987, Medical Management Group of New York, Inc. has provided appointment services for over 500,000 Independent Medical Examinations (IMEs), Independent Medical Record Reviews (IMRs), Peer Reviews, and Radiology Reviews. In addition, we provide corresponding Medical Record Retrieval services. Our core of competency includes General Liability, Auto, No-Fault, Workers' Compensation, and Disability claims."

# # #
Medical Mutual
Medical Mutual
http://www.medmutual.com
http://twitter.com/medmutual

"Medical Mutual is the oldest and largest health insurer in Ohio."

# # #
Medical Review Institute of America (MRIoA)
Medical Review Institute of America (MRIoA)
http://www.mrioa.com
file reviews

"Medical Review Institute of America, Inc. (MRIoA) was incorporated in 1983. Today MRIoA is an industry leader in providing external review resources for over 800 clients nationwide. MRIoA provides review of medical, dental, behavioral health, pharmacy, vision, disability, workers' compensation, and auto claims for insurance carriers, employers, TPAs, self- administered union groups, pharmacy benefit managers, human resource consultants and departments of insurance throughout the country. MRIoA utilizes a nationwide network of board-certified physician specialists and professionals in over 133 specialties and sub-specialties of medicine. MRIoA also has reviewers in most states, offering the most extensive same-state reviewer resources available from an external review organization. MRIoA holds dual accreditation with URAC with certificates in Health Utilization Management and as an Independent Review Organization. In addition we are NCQA and SSAE 16 certified.

MRIoA's goal is to render a professional, independent and unbiased opinion to assist our clients with their adjudication challenges or to provide an external source to comply with ERISA/DOL or state laws.

MRIoA reviews cases prospectively, concurrently and retrospectively for: Medical Necessity, Appropriate Treatment, Experimental Procedures, Utilization Frequency, Appropriate Hospitalization, Formulary Criteria Review, Pre-Existing Conditions, Injury Causation, CPT Coding, Level of Disability, Provider Fees, Outpatient Facility Fees, and all Diagnostic Testing and Charges.

MRIoA has provided state-level external review in many states since 2001. MRIoA is also contracted with hundreds of clients to offer Federal External Review under the ACA."

# # #
Medical Review Stream (Concentra)
Medical Review Stream (Concentra)
http://www.concentra.com/employers/consulting/medical-reviewstream/
file reviews

"With so many new options for peer review services, it's important to be selective when choosing a medical peer review provider. Medical ReviewStream™ by Concentra can help you resolve complex or contested workers' compensation claims using board-certified physicians who offer a wide breadth of specialties. We provide pharmacy reviews, utilization reviews, complex chart reviews, Family Medical Leave Act (FMLA) Reviews, disability reviews, and claims adjudication services in a timely and cost-efficient manner.

Our medical opinion review services can not only help you contain medical costs, but also streamline your utilization review process, provide the Medical Advisor coverage you need, and help you ensure compliance with URAC, HIPAA and jurisdictional requirements. Medical ReviewStream™ is accredited by the URAC in Workers' Compensation Utilization Management. All reviews are performed in accordance with state-mandated requirements or URAC standards, whichever are more stringent.

As an industry leader, our knowledge, experience, and technology provides reliable evaluations through an extensive panel of expert Medical Advisors."

# # #
Medical Systems, inc....
Medical Systems, inc.
http://www.medicalsystemsusa.com/
http://twitter.com/MedSystemsUSA
IME and file reviews

"Medical Systems is a partner in our clients' success. In providing INDEPENDENT Medical Evaluations (IMEs) to our clients, we strive to anticipate their needs through total engagement – every Medical Systems team member focuses on ensuring you receive a credible report, timely report as efficiently and cost-effectively as possible.

How do we accomplish this? We are resolute in our commitment to excellence and independence. Our schedulers take pride in finding the best doctor options for even the most complicated and unusual claims. Doctors routinely laud our records department for how efficiently the medical records are organized. Our QA department strives to ensure all reports are consistent and notifies you in advance when the result is unexpected. But we do not rest there. We offer education opportunities to our clients through our annual symposium, restaurant-based luncheon programs, and customized on-site learning opportunities.

Medical Systems also believes in and adheres to the idea that IMEs should be independent. That is why we are a privately held corporation without exclusive contracts with any doctor. We know that credibility is the most important quality in any IME report. And no IME report can be credible unless it is truly independent."

# # #
Medilex
Medilex
http://www.medilexinc.com/
expert witness

"Medilex experts are available to review materials, consult with attorneys, prepare written reports, work on affidavits, and provide expert testimony."

# # #

Medinsights (Gallagher Bassett Services)
Medinsights (Gallagher Bassett Services)
http://www.medinsights.com/

"MedInsights offers individualized, managed medical care services to insured and self-insured companies.

Services include:

Field Case Management
Telephonic Case Management
Utilization Management
Pharmacy Benefits Management
Medical Bill Management
Medical Legal Review
Medicare Secondary Payer Compliance & Resolution
Occupational Health Consulting Services"

# # #
MedManagement
MedManagement
> http://www.medmanagementllc.com/
> file reviews

"MedManagement, LLC was founded in 1995 to provide clinical and financial management tools and resources to providers. With a keen eye toward the ever-changing healthcare regulatory landscape, we identify the needs of health care providers and insurers, responding with valuable services and meaningful insights. MedManagement, LLC remains the corporate parent of EdiPhy Advisors."

# # #
Mednick Associates
Mednick Associates
http://www.mednickassociates.com/
info@mednickassociates.com

"We are always looking for physicians to help review
the SSA disability appeals cases in the specialties of
psych, ortho and internal med. This is non clinical
sidework that is flexible in nature and can be done
around your schedule."
Erinn Crane, BSN, RN | Medical Expert Coordinator |
203.966.3000 (o)Ext. 117 | Fax 203.745.2007
erinn@mednickassociates.com | 400 N. Main Ste. 200M,
Davenport, IA 52801

# # #
MedQuest Evaluators http://medquest.imebase.com
MedQuest Evaluators
      http://medquest.imebase.com
      IME
      amy@medquestevaluatorsime.com

"We schedule Independent Medical Exams for
employers regarding workers' compensation, fitness for
duty and short term disability."

# # #
MedReview (NYCHSRO) http://web.medreview.us/
MedReview (NYCHSRO) http://web.medreview.us/
hr@medreview.us

"New York County Health Services Review Organization (NYCHSRO) was founded as a 501 (c) (3) not-for-profit corporation in 1974 under the Federal Law mandating Professional Standards Review Organizations (PSROs) for Medicare and Medicaid review. In 2013, NYCHSRO is observing its thirty-ninth (39th) year of continuous active service in medical review in New York State.

MedReview, Inc. is a wholly owned subsidiary of NYCHSRO, and a for-profit corporation, formed in 1984 to offer utilization management and analysis services to the private sector, including labor organizations, corporations, insurance companies, and managed care organizations.

NYCHSRO/MedReview's mission is to provide health care assessment services that assist clients in improving the appropriateness, quality, and cost-effectiveness of health care.

NYCHSRO/MedReview has a well-established reputation in medical reviews and in programs for prospective, concurrent and retrospective monitoring. It is dedicated to working with clients to tailor review programs specific to their needs, corporate philosophy, and benefit structure. In the era of increased reliance on managed care, NYCHSRO/MedReview provides its clients with guaranteed cost-effective case management and utilization analysis approaches that can assist them in developing more cost-effective benefit plan strategies.

NYCHSRO/MedReview is governed by a Board of Directors, and is administered by its Chief Executive Officer, Joseph B. Stamm, who reports to the Board. NYCHSRO/MedReview's senior staff is comprised of an Executive Vice President/Chief Financial Officer, Senior Vice President/Chief Operating Officer, five (5) Vice Presidents and a Chief Medical Officer. NYCHSRO/MedReview has a staff of more than 200 full-time employees.

NYCHSRO/MedReview was among the first organizations registered as a certified Utilization Review (UR) agent in New York when UR registration began in 1997 and it achieved PRO-like entity status in 1995. That designation was updated to a QIO-like entity in 2008. The QIO-like entity status means that NYCHSRO/MedReview is a physician-access organization that has:

Access to doctors of medicine or osteopathy, licensed and practicing in the State, to conduct review for the organization,

Availability of at least one physician, licensed in the State, from every generally recognized specialty and subspecialty who is actively practicing in the area they review, and

NYCHSRO/MedReview is not a health care facility, health care facility association, or health care facility affiliate.

NYCHSRO/MedReview is accredited by URAC as an Independent Review Organization (IRO) and as a Health Utilization Management (HUM) organization. NYCHSRO/MedReview only uses medical professionals who are licensed and registered in their specific disciplines. Over the past twenty years, NYCHSRO/MedReview has conducted over 2 million peer reviews to evaluate clinical decisions and services rendered by medical practitioners at all levels of the health care continuum. NYCHSRO/MedReview maintains a physician review panel of more than 100 clinicians, in 74 specialties and subspecialties. Presently, NYCHSRO/MedReview has its headquarters in New York City, with a new office recently established in Massachusetts. As NYCHSRO/MedReview's services are provided around the country, it is anticipated that additional offices will be established to facilitate provision of service to those local markets.

For inquiries about job openings, please send an email to: hr@medreview.us

# # #
MedRisk
MedRisk
http://www.medrisknet.com

"MedRisk is a leading provider of managed physical medicine and diagnostic imaging services for the workers' compensation industry and related markets."

# # #
MedSource National

MedSource National

http://www.medsourceime.com/
https://twitter.com/medsourcenation
IME and file reviews
ime@msnime.com

"MedSource National is an affiliate company of MedSource Services Inc., a Michigan-based, Independent Medical Exam (IME) and Review firm servicing the Midwest since 1993.

As a result of the rapid, nationwide consolidation of the claims, healthcare review and IME industries, the need arose for a firm that was stable, integrated and ready to deliver accurate information to insurance carriers, employers, and third party administrators on a national level.

MedSource National was established to fill this need; to build upon and apply to the national claims market the personal, regional service that had made MedSource Services Inc. successful for two decades.

Med Source National currently maintains offices in Michigan, New York and Florida, with client management contacts who live and work in New York, California, Illinois, Michigan, Florida, Maryland, Arizona and Massachusetts. Because we assist our clients with claims in across the country, MedSource National maintains a panel of credentialed IME and Peer Review providers in all 50 states."

# # #
MedWatch
MedWatch
http://www.urmedwatch.com/

"MedWatch is a full-spectrum care management company providing clinical risk management solutions to the self-funded health plan market since 1988. Our programs are built on the philosophy that assertive, professional and personalized healthcare management should meet the clinical needs of clients and their employees while also performing cost containment support of the plan.

MedWatch proudly maintains triple URAC accreditation, further demonstrating it's commitment to quality health care; MedWatch current accreditations: MedWatch

Health Utilization Management since 1997
Case Management since 2000
Population Health Management since 2007"

# # #
MedWork
MedWork
http://www.medwork.org/

"Medwork of Wisconsin, Inc. is an Independent Review Organization that specializes in medical necessity and experimental treatment issues. Medwork provides high quality reviews that are free from conflict of interest for healthcare entities that require a neutral third-party opinion.

Reviews are fair and impartial and benefit both the provider and the patient. Medwork helps to improve the quality of medicine and enhance healthcare, ensuring healthcare services are provided in the most appropriate manner possible.

Medwork provides independent, external reviews that assist insurance payors, state regulatory agencies, and medical and claims managers achieve cost control and provide the right care for each patient."

# # #
Memorial Hermann...
Memorial Hermann
http://healthplan.memorialhermann.org
Health Insurance in Houston

# # #
MES Solutions
MES Solutions
https://www.messolutions.com
        IME and file reviews
        info@messolutions.com
"MES Solutions (MES) was founded in 1978 and was one of the first companies established to provide the claims community access to physicians with expertise in conducting Independent Medical Examinations, Peer, Record, and Bill Reviews."

# # #
MESSA
MESSA
http://www.messa.org

"In 1937, the Michigan Education Association started the first group hospitalization program for school employees. That program evolved through the years and the Michigan Education Special Services Association (MESSA) was formed in 1960. We are a not-for-profit voluntary employees' beneficiary association (VEBA). Since 1965, Michigan educators have collectively bargained their benefits with employers.

Today, MESSA is a leader in the Michigan education market, providing outstanding personal customer service and comprehensive medical and prescription coverage, large networks and doctor choice. We also offer vision, dental and short-term and long-term disability benefits. Our members include teachers, education support professionals, K-12 administrators and higher education faculty and staff."

# # #
Met Healthcare Solutions
Met Healthcare Solutions http://www.met-hcs.com/
IME and file reviews

"MET Healthcare Solutions, a URAC accredited IRO, specializes in Independent Medical Reviews (IRO), Texas Designated Doctor Services, and Independent Medical Evaluations (IME). MET has over 20 years of experience recruiting and credentialing physicians and healthcare providers across the nation to meet the geographic requirements of our clients. Our national medical expert panel of healthcare providers are board certified and trained to perform independent medical reviews, independent medical examinations, medical consultations, Texas designated doctor examinations, diagnostic testing, and other healthcare related services nationwide."

# # #
MetLife
MetLife
http://www.metlife.com
http://twitter.com/metlife
They have file review opportunities including opportunities as in-house file reviewers on disability claims.

# # #
MHM Services
MHM Services
http://www.mhm-services.com/

"MHM Provides behavioral health and medical specialty services to governmental agencies in a wide variety of patient care settings, Including correctional facilities, state hospitals, courts, juvenile facilities and community clinics."

# # #
MHN
MHN
http://www.mhn.com

"MHN's products range from Employee Assistance Programs (EAPs) and behavioral health services to organizational development and wellness programs. MHN's solutions promote work/life balance, wellness, employee productivity and organizational efficiency. MHN and its affiliated companies provide EAP, non-medical counseling, behavioral health care and other services through commercial, affiliate and government accounts. With over 30 years of behavioral health care experience, MHN serves over 1,200 client accounts, including Fortune 500 companies, government agencies, multi-employer funds and affiliate accounts through Health Net.

MHN partners with a nationwide provider network of over 55,000 licensed practitioners and 1,400 hospitals and care facilities.

MHN also partners and collaborates with leading behavioral health organizations to promote best practices and add to the awareness of behavioral health issues, including the Association for Behavioral Health and Wellness (ABHW), the Council for Affordable Quality Healthcare (CAQH), and the California Association of Health Plans (CAHP).

MHN is URAC accredited in Health Utilization Management and Health Network and is licensed under the Knox-Keene Health Care Service Plan Act as a specialized health care service plan in mental health and chemical dependency.
Headquartered in San Rafael, California, MHN has offices and call centers throughout the United States."

# # #
MHNet
MHNet
http://www.mhnet.com/

"MHNet is a national behavioral health care company headquartered in Austin, TX. Founded by clinicians in 1985, we offer a comprehensive suite of behavioral health products for employers, health plans and public programs."

# # #
MHS Health Wisconsin
MHS Health Wisconsin
www.mhswi.com
https://twitter.com/MHS_Wisconsin

"Wisconsin-based MHS Health is a managed care company that employs more than 140 people in our Milwaukee office. MHS Health is a wholly owned subsidiary of Centene Corporation, a leading multi-line healthcare enterprise offering both core Medicaid and specialty services. MHS Health is licensed by the Wisconsin Office of Insurance and is a Qualified Health Plan issuer in the Wisconsin Health Insurance Marketplace."

# # #
Michigan IME (Michigan)
Michigan IME (Michigan) http://michiganime.com/
Info@michiganime.com

MICHIGAN IME,
we are located in Madison Heights MI. Our address is 939 E 12 Mile Road, Madison Heights MI 48071. Lastly, thank yo so much for thinking of us.

· Who can providers contact to discuss working with your organization (and how should they contact them)? THEY CAN CONTACT US DIRECTLY AT 248-939-8235 OR VIA EMAIL AT pwebster@michiganime.com
· Which types of health care providers do you recruit? For example, do you recruit only physicians or do you also recruit psychologists, chiropractors and other disciplines. WE RECRUIT CHIRO'S AND NEUROPSYCHS AND EVERY OTHER SPECIALTY.

· What types of services do you tend to offer in relation to medical records reviews and/or IME's? WE OFFER CLIENTS RECORD REVIEWS, IME'S, FMLA'S 2ND AND 3RD OPINIONS AND OCCASIONALLY PEER RIEWS

· Do your opportunities require the professional to be in active clinical practice and if so how is active clinical practice defined (ex: number of hours per week/ percentage of income from direct treatment)? ANY PRACTIONERS NEED TO BE AT 30% TREATING

· What opportunities, if any, do you have for professionals who are not currently in active clinical practice? JUST FOR REVIEW OF RECORDS OR PEERS

· Are you recruiting providers on a nationwide level or are there particular areas of the country you work in (if so which areas of the country are you currently recruiting in)? RIGHT NOW WE ARE PRIMARILY MICHIGAN DR.S WITH OCCASIONAL DR.S IN OH AND IN ILL BUT THAT IS A SMALL AMOUNT.

· Do you have a description of your company and what you do that you'd like to have included in the company directory of the book? WE DO

· If possible (and it is understandable if you can't), can you estimate what you typically pay to consultants or otherwise describe as much about how consultants are paid as possible? OUR EXPERTS ARE PAID 30 DAYS FROM RECEIPT OF THE FINISHED REPORT AND WE WORK WITH DR.S AND CLINICIANS ON WHAT THERE REQUIRED FEES ARE. THERE ARE NO SET FEES.

Michigan IME
P: 248.565.8235
F: 248.565.8398
info@michiganime.com
www.michiganime.com

# # #
Mid Atlantic Health Solutions
Mid Atlantic Health Solutions
http://www.mahsolutions.com/

"Mid Atlantic Health Solutions is a for-profit, limited liability company in southeast Virginia offering Utilization Management, Case Management, Maternity Management, and Diabetes Management services to self- funded health plans. We also offer credentialing solutions for independent physician practices and group medical practices. Our Utilization Management services provide telephonic medical necessity reviews for prospective, concurrent, and retrospective cases on a national level. Mid Atlantic Health Solutions processes are based upon nationally recognized standards, evaluated by a comprehensive quality management program, and measured for effectiveness against industry benchmarks. Case Management, Maternity Management, and Diabetes Management Programs complement the Utilization Management services offered. Simple Solutions, our physician credentialing service, assists individual physicians as well as larger group practices in navigating the credentialing process required by health plans/networks and hospitals for participation."

###
Mitchell
Mitchell
http://www.mitchell.com/
http://twitter.com/Mitchell_Intl

"Mitchell was born out of a desire to meet the practical demands of the automotive industry, delivering the industry's first accurate, fu33nctioning car parts replacement resource for collision-damaged vehicles. Our focus on simplification, efficiency and access to accurate information, drove our entry first into the collision repair market and then into auto physical damage claims.

Since then, we have extended our solution offering beyond collision repair and auto physical damage claims to include auto casualty, workers' compensation, and pharmacy claims handling. Today, we empower clients across the Property and Casualty industry by providing them with smart technology solutions, deep industry expertise, and seamless connections to the broadest range of solutions, networks, and partners."

###
MLS Group of Companies (MLS)...
MLS Group of Companies (MLS)
https://www.mls-ime.com/
IME and file reviews
info@mls-ime.com

"The MLS Group of Companies (MLS) is a leading URAC accredited national provider of Peer Review Services, Independent Medical Evaluations, FMLA Medical Assessments and Functional Capacity Evaluations. Our accredited national network of physicians and allied medical professionals service the entire United States. MLS is recognized for our experience and commitment to providing exceptional client service, objective medical assessments, and the protections associated with cutting edge information technology. A trademark of MLS is the extensive involvement of all medical staff, coordinators, administrators and senior management. We provide efficient, cost-effective service by selecting team members with appropriate skills and experience to handle the needs of all parties involved for effective claims resolution."

# # #

MMRO (Managed Medical Review Organization)
MMRO (Managed Medical Review Organization)
http://www.mmroinc.com/
file reviews

"Since our inception in 2007, MMRO has been a leader in providing clients with disability claims management and medical review services that help improve organizations performance through effective people, superior administration, and industry standards. Our solutions are shaped by each client's unique needs and designed to ensure superior quality, credibility, and reliable innovation. MMRO clients consist of public employee retirement systems, employers, third party administrators, insurance companies, and government agencies seeking to promote positive outcomes while controlling administrative and benefit costs."

###
Moonlight Exams
Moonlight Exams
http://www.moonlightexams.com

# # #
Mountain-Pacific Quality Health http://mpqhf.com/
Mountain-Pacific Quality Health
    http://mpqhf.com/

"Mountain-Pacific Quality Health is a nonprofit corporation that strives to be the "go-to" resource for driving innovation in health care systems in the states and territories we serve. We first began partnering with providers, practitioners and patients in Montana in 1973. With four decades of experience, we now support the health care communities of Montana, Wyoming, Hawaii, Alaska, Guam, American Samoa and the Commonwealth of the Northern Mariana Islands."

# # #
MPRO
MPRO
http://www.mpro.org/
http://twitter.com/MPROcares
file reviews

"MPRO is a nonprofit organization and national leader in healthcare quality improvement and medical review. Our goal is simple - we are helping healthcare get better. MPRO provides medical consulting and review, as well as data analysis to federal agencies, state Medicaid and public health organizations, healthcare facilities, private health plans and other third party payers. In addition, MPRO represents Michigan in Lake Superior Quality Innovation Network (QIN), which also serves Minnesota and Wisconsin under the Centers for Medicare & Medicaid Services (CMS) Quality Improvement Organization (QIO) Program.

MPRO is committed to improving the quality, safety and efficiency of healthcare. Although we do not see patients, we are healthcare professionals (including physicians and nurses) and consultants who work with healthcare providers to promote the adoption and use of evidence-based best practices and processes to achieve our healthcare quality goals. Our services offer our clients and partners access to a proven, impartial, connected resource that understands the intricacies of healthcare. It is our #1 priority to provide thoughtful evidence-based strategies and solutions that help them achieve their healthcare quality improvement goals and outcomes."

# # #
MRG exams
MRG exams
http://www.mrgexams.com/
IME's
JoinOurPanel@MRGexams.com

"MRG Exams has opportunities for physicians to perform independent medical exams and peer reviews as a complement to your existing medical practice. Our ongoing training and education is valued by our physicians as they continue their growth as independent evaluators.

As a service company we simplify the exam process by handling the administrative tasks, allowing you to do what you do best. Our quality management team works with you to ensure that all reports are clear, concise and that your opinions are well supported."

# # #
MSLA
MSLA
http://www.mslaca.com/services/disability-insurance-tpa-services.php
file reviews, IME, VA

"MSLA was established in 1998 and has been growing ever since. We have built our reputation on superior customer service, outstanding report quality, and rapid turnaround time. Our business philosophy incorporates exceptional customer service and accurate evaluations, both of which are the primary factors for our growth since our inception."

# # #
Mutual of Omaha http://www.mutualofomaha.com/
Mutual of Omaha
http://www.mutualofomaha.com/
http://twitter.com/mutualofomaha

"For more than a century, Mutual of Omaha has been committed to helping our customers through life's transitions by providing an array of insurance, financial and banking products."

# # #
National Claim Evaluations...
National Claim Evaluations
http://www.natclaim.com/
IME and file reviews   natclaim@natclaim.com

"NCEI is a value added provider of IME and related solutions without the high price associated with service intensive boutiques. Founded in 1985, NCEI is a pioneer in the IME industry. As an industry pioneer, NCEI made the decision not to follow the growth path of many of its competitors. Instead of developing into a large inflexible impersonal provider, we chose to develop and occupy a value added position in the marketplace. This positioning has been rewarded by the marketplace. Many clients are seeking a high touch approach to the IME process, in addition to support with using medical data to reduce claim and fraud costs. National Claim Evaluations is designed for and built to serve this client."

# # #
National Imaging Associates
National Imaging Associates
http://www1.radmd.com/
http://www.niahealthcare.com/

"Welcome to National Imaging Associates (NIA), your trusted partner in clinical decision support. As a pioneer in the radiology benefits management industry, we have delivered innovative solutions to effectively manage the cost and quality of advanced medical imaging since 1995. These solutions translate into powerful results for our health plan and government agency customers, as well as their providers and consumers.

With NIA's long-standing experience, our team's unmatched clinical expertise, and the backing of our parent organization, Magellan Health, Inc., we bring more power to you than anyone else in the industry.

Tap into the power of our long-time history and experience. Let us anticipate tomorrow's problems and opportunities to help you stay ahead of the curve. Draw power from NIA's market leadership. From our market-leading data analytics and the industry's most experienced team of professionals, to the most thorough provider privileging standards and consumer awareness outreach, NIA continues to lead the way. Utilize insightful research, conducted by NIA's clinical experts, to empower your business, your providers and your consumers through informed choices, optimal outcomes and predictable results.
You can expect all of this from NIA, plus the power of flexible solutions, specifically designed to meet your strategic business needs. That's the power of NIA. More power to you."

# # #
National Independent Review Organization (NIRO)
National Independent Review Organization (NIRO)
http://iniro.com
file review

"NIRO provides independent unbiased medical reviews in all specialties. The medical reviews are conducted by experienced board certified physicians, who are dedicated to providing our clients with prompt, accurate, and unbiased medical reviews."

# # #
National Medical Consultants/National Medical...
National Medical Consultants/National Medical Examiners
http://www.nationalmedicalconsultants.com/
IME and file reviews
medicalconsultants@nyc.rr.com

"National Medical Consultants, P.C. is a physician owned and operated company representing a panel of over 3700 medical experts who are distinguished specialists in all areas of medicine.

Our physicians do not consider themselves to be a part of a service but a group of doctors from some of the finest institutions giving honest objective opinions in medical malpractice cases for both the plaintiff and defense."

# # #
National Medical Reviews (NMR)...
National Medical Reviews (NMR)
http://nationalmedicalreviews.com/
file reviews and IME
medreviews@nmrusa.com

"NMR's panel consists of 500 individual providers, representing over 700 board certifications, specialties and state licenses nationwide."

"NMR's clients include health insurers, managed care organizations, health maintenance organizations, preferred provider organizations, third party administrators, multi-employer and self-funded plans, federally regulated entities, medical and utilization management firms, workers' compensation carriers, state labor and industry departments, departments of public health, Department of Justice, hospitals, law firms and other medical review companies."

# # #
Network Medical Review co (NMR) [an ExamWorks co]
Network Medical Review co (NMR) [an ExamWorks co]
      https://www.nmrco.com/
IME and file reviews

"NMR is an Independent Review Organization that specializes in Evidence-Based Medical solutions for the insurance, managed care, legal and medical industries. Board Certified Specialists offer fair and consistent evaluations of a full spectrum of medical conditions."

# # #
New Century Health...
New Century Health
      http://www.newcenturyhealth.com/
      ghabeych@newcenturyhealth.com

"To deliver specialty care management solutions that leverage technology and evidence-based medicine at the point-of-care, with a focus on oncology and cardiology. Our services promote the most effective treatment, reduce variability, improve clinical outcomes, and optimize cost-effectiveness."

# # #
New Directions
New Directions
http://www.ndbh.com

"We offer a full range of behavioral health solutions. Our relationship with health plans enables us to integrate our services seamlessly with traditional medical support. Our managed behavioral health services include incisive analytics, the finest in quality assurance and customer service that goes beyond the extra mile in providing care."

# # #
New England Medical Legal Consultants...
New England Medical Legal Consultants
        http://www.nemlc.com/
        Expert witness; legal/malpractice
        consultants@nemlc.com
1507 Post Road   ; Warwick, RI 02888
(401) 352-0088

# # #
New York Medical Management (NYMM)...
New York Medical Management (NYMM)
        http://www.nymm.org/

"New York Medical Management (NYMM) has been providing Medical Review and Utilization Management services to insurance companies, Independent Practice Associations (IPA), Preferred Provider Networks (PPO) and self-insured, self-administered health plans for the past fifteen years."

# # #
NextCare Health http://www.nextcarehealth.com/...
NextCare Health   http://www.nextcarehealth.com/
             https://twitter.com/NEXtCAREHealth
Middle East, etc.

"We are the leading Third Party Administrator in the MENA region, recognized by our customers as providers of quality services; we will continuously work on improving them, growing into new markets and upholding our core values and commitments, while continuously maintaining our high standards.

We maintain a continued focus on our customers and their changing needs, by listening and conducting ongoing reviews of our customer service approach. We periodically review our internal processes in order to maximize efficiency of claims authorization and processing. We keep our systems up-to-date as part of our integrated solutions to clients ensuring that we are leaders within this field."

# # #
Nexus Medical Consulting

Nexus Medical Consulting
       http://nexmc.com
       https://twitter.com/nexusmedical
IME and file reviews
(affiliated with ProPeer Resources)

"Nexus Medical has set the standard for excellence for independent reviews. Nexus specializes in providing various types of medical reviews to many nationally recognized/accredited healthcare providers and law firms. Nexus has a reputation with our clients for delivering reliable excellence in the shortest amount of time. Our competency is proven to serve our clients' needs and enables our physicians to be more productive while increasing their report accuracy and quality."

"Nexus is an efficient, adaptive and independent Utilization Review Company that takes pride in delivering reliable excellence. We provide quality utilization and specialty peer reviews, along with many other legal and exam services. We were founded in 2009 and have recently been recognized as a member of Inc.'s 5,000 fastest growing companies in 2015. Nexus is a fully URAC accredited U/R company serving clients in all 50 states, as well as Puerto Rico and United Arab Emirates. Our corporate headquarters is located in Central Texas, however, we have a broad review panel of over 550 physicians licensed throughout the country. All are board certified, thoroughly screened and credentialed. Our network of doctors work with group health plans, worker's compensation, self-funded employers, TPA's and legal professionals to connect quality with outcomes. Our diverse panel covers 85+ specialties to meet any medical review needs that you may have.

Review Services Nexus Medical is proud to offer:

- Medical Necessity Reviews
- Work Comp Reviews
- Group Health Reviews
- Pre-Authorization Reviews
- Post-Service Retrospective Reviews
- Appeal Reviews
- PPACA and ERISA Reviews
- Drug Utilization Reviews
- Pharmacy Reviews
- Continuation of Care Plans

- Vocational Consulting
- Complex/Legacy/Peer Reviews
- Standard of Care Reviews
- Experimental/Investigational Reviews
- Retrospective & Concurrent Length of Stay Reviews
- Diagnostic Testing Reviews
- Specialty Reviews including IRO
- Long Term/Short Term Disability Reviews
- Auto Liability Reviews
- CPT Code/Billing Reviews
- Hospital Bill Review, Re-Pricing and Audits
- Expert Testimony
- Cost Projection Analysis
- Medical Legal Reviews
- Functional Capacity Evaluations
- Independent Medical Exams (IME)"

Nexus reports having a lot of different types of reviews but much of what they do are cases with a requested same day turnaround time. One of the services Nexus offers is utilization reviews to determine whether a treatment is medically necessary. Nexus has a utilization review nurse summarize the case to help the medical consultant. They note that these streamlined cases tend to take 15 to 20 minutes and they ask for a quick turnaround of just a few hours. For some things they'd like you to be in active practice which they defined as at least 20 hours per week.

Nexus tends to ask for an exclusivity contract--- meaning that any companies that your work with first through them you can only work with through them.

# # #
North American Consultants...
North American Consultants
www.northamericanconsultants.com

# # #
Northern Ohio Medical Management Corp (NOMMC)
Northern Ohio Medical Management Corp (NOMMC)
http://www.nommc.com/
IME and file reviews
info@nommc.com

"We are expanding our Physician Network of Board Certified Physicians nationwide."
# # #

Northwood
Northwood
http://www.northwoodinc.com
info@northwoodinc.com

"Northwood, Inc. was established in 1992 as a specialized network of durable medical equipment, prosthetics, orthotics and medical supplies (DMEPOS) providers offering cost-effective, high-quality products to health plans and self-funded groups.

Northwood has been listening to the needs of our auto and workers' compensation clients and has applied its provider network techniques to other necessary service lines to effectively manage the care of an injured claimant."

# # #
Objective Medical Assessments Corporation (OMAC)...
Objective Medical Assessments Corporation (OMAC)
https://www.omacime.com
physicianrelations@omacime.com

# # #
OccuCare (Teamhealth)
OccuCare (Teamhealth)
        Ohio; Pennsylvania
        http://occucareime.com
IME

"Occucare's primary service is performing Independent Medical Evaluations (IMEs). These IMEs may be conducted for a variety of medical or legal reasons, such as when a claimant exhibits one or more disabilities that appear to be due to job-related accidents or illnesses.

As an independent, non-treating physician group, Occucare offers its clients:

An impartial and neutral evaluation of the claimant, thus eliminating "conflict-of-interest" issues that a clinical physician may encounter
The convenience of scheduling assessments via phone, email or on-line
A roster of quality physicians with diverse specialties
Expertly written, standardized physician reports
State-of-the-art transcription service that produces quality, timely reports within days of the examination

Rush/Stat file reviews

A medical–legal expert who is available on request to discuss the IME report

A medical review officer

A registered pharmacist

Exceptional customer service

Occucare has been providing IME service to risk management companies, MCOs, TPAs, Workers' Compensation consultants, self-insured employers, legal firms and insurance companies across the country since 1988.

Our clients can feel confident in the knowledge that our credentialed physicians are experienced in their specialty and provide complete, objective and accurate IME reports. Occucare physicians are experienced with and strictly follow the criteria as set forth in: the AMA Guides to the Evaluation of Permanent Impairment, 5th Edition in determining impairment, disability and handicap; the ODG Treatment Guidelines when assessing treatment issues; the Miller components when considering medical necessity; and Mercy Guidelines when determining Chiropractic issues."

# # #

Occupational Health Link (Ohio)...

Occupational Health Link (Ohio)

http://www.oehpmco.com/

"As your Managed Care Organization, Occupational Health Link's mission is to provide workers' compensation and occupational health solutions through ethical medical systems and state-of-the art information systems built on a philosophy that "Work is Part of Healing." We are a medium size MCO, serving approximately 9,000 employers. We are dedicated to individualized assistance and one-on-one contact. Our commitment to quality includes a pledge to provide local/regional medical management for the injured worker – we're close by when you need us!"

# # #
OFMQ
OFMQ
http://www.ofmq.com/

"OFMQ is a healthcare consulting services company. Since 1972, we've been committed to advancing the quality of healthcare and improving lives. As an independent not-for-profit organization, our service lines include quality improvement, health information technology, data analytics and health care review.

What We Do/Our Mission: Our focus is to lead efforts to improve health care and improve lives. OFMQ is the essential, recognized resource and innovative expert in healthcare quality and improving outcomes through:

Accelerating research into practice;
Engaging and collaborating with communities;
Advancing the implementation and use of health information technology;

Achieving improvements in health quality;
Empowering consumers to make informed health
decisions."

# # #
OHARA
OHARA
http://www.oharallc.com/

"OHARA is an established managed care company in
Sioux Falls, South Dakota. OHARA opened its' doors in
January of 1995 as a limited liability company. OHARA
has focused to meet the managed care needs of
insurance carriers specializing in workers'
compensation. In January 1997, services were
established for the group health market. In December
1998, OHARA became URAC accredited in the areas of
Health Utilization Management Standards and
Workers' Compensation Utilization Management
Standards and we achieved URAC accreditation in
Case Management in 2005. OHARA continues to be
accredited in Case Management and Workers'
Compensation Utilization Management We are
presently located in Cherapa Place, a certified "green"
building on the East Bank of the Big Sioux River in
downtown Sioux Falls.

OHARA offers a full spectrum of services to insurance carriers, third party administrators and self-insured employers in the Midwest region. These services now include: Case Management for workers' compensation injuries, Preferred Provider Organizations, Bill Review, Vocational Rehabilitation, Life Care Planning and Pharmacy Benefit Programs. This service area has expanded to include the states of Colorado, Iowa, Kansas and Missouri. In Minnesota, services include case management and vocational rehabilitation for workers' compensation injuries.

OHARA is committed to providing professional managed care services to insurance carriers, third party administrators and self-insured employers in the Midwest."

# # #
OMCA
OMCA
http://www.omca.biz/
https://twitter.com/OMCAInc

"As the first MCO approved in Kentucky, OMCA has remained a leader in providing innovative costs containment solutions. Managing workers' compensation expense has become increasingly difficult in the environment of rapidly escalating medical costs. Payors constantly struggle with excessive medical expenses while providing quality medical care for injured workers.

Aggressive medical management by select occupational healthcare professionals is critical in achieving cost efficient, optimal outcomes. OMCA products represent years of experience, innovation and collaborative relationships with our select physician panel.
OMCA arranges and conducts a variety of seminars for our customers and clients. These seminars cover a variety of workers' compensation, ethics and medical cost containment topics."

# # #
OmniMed Evaluation Services http://omnimed.net/
OmniMed Evaluation Services
> http://omnimed.net/
IME and file reviews

# # #
Oncology Analytics...
Oncology Analytics
> http://www.oncologyanalytics.com

# # #
One America
One America
http://www.oneamerica.com
https://twitter.com/OneAmerica

"In a world where stability has increasing value, especially for financial services companies, you can count on the companies of OneAmerica®. We have built a 135-year foundation of strength, and we will continue to thrive and grow by keeping our commitments to stability and ongoing policyholder value.

Among our financial company peers, we continue to outperform. We have become one of the fastest-growing mutual insurance companies in the U.S. Today, the companies of OneAmerica rely on a national network of financial professionals to provide customers with products and services:

Retirement products and services
Individual life insurance and annuities
Asset-based long-term care
Employee benefits"

###
OpinionEx
OpinionEx
https://www.opinionex.com
Expert witness directory

# # #
Optum
Optum
www.optum.com
https://twitter.com/optum

"Optum® is a health services and innovation company."

# # #
OrthoNet
OrthoNet
http://www.orthonet-online.com/
utilization review
1311 Mamaroneck Avenue; Suite 240   White Plains, NY 10605
800-372-8922

"OrthoNet is the leading orthopaedic specialty benefit management company in the United States. Our innovative care management model integrates the needs of providers, payors, and members to ensure the delivery of high quality, cost-effective care while realizing substantial savings that keep the costs of healthcare down."

# # #
P&S Network http://www.pandsnetwork.com
P&S Network   http://www.pandsnetwork.com
        file review

"Independent Review

Independent medical peer review services are at the core of our business. The purpose of these reviews is to help keep health care costs down and also to ensure that patients receive appropriate medical treatment. P&S currently offers IRO services for multiple states and insurance companies. The rising cost of healthcare effects everyone. The IRO process helps avoid unnecessary repetitive appeals and provides a conflict-free determination performed by specialty-matched board certified physicians, which can then be utilized to resolve medical treatment disputes.

Workers Compensation UR Determinations

Since 2003, P&S Network has provided high quality peer reviews for competitive prices for carriers, third party administrators, utilization review organizations, and employers. Our difference is that we offer one point of contact, accessible during business hours for all time zones within the U.S. You will find that our staff are knowledgeable and can accommodate your specifications for the report. This quality staff ensures excellent reports and fast turn-around times. We offer highly competitive pricing, as well as next day turn around to help you meet your demanding deadlines. Same day stat reporting is also available if needed. We have an extensive panel of physicians, all of whom are board certified in their respective specialties. We offer state matching when required or requested.

Pharmacy and Medications Peer Reviews

P&S Network is one of the pioneers in identifying the explosion of use of high cost prescription drugs in workers compensation and executing innovative solutions to ensure the safe and cost effective use of medications. With our extensive knowledge of evidence-based pain management, we work with treating physicians to assist them in discontinuing patients from risky levels of opioids/narcotics. Your costs are reduced when we identify drugs that should not be billed through workers comp and obtain agreements from providers to substitute generics for expensive brand name drugs. You will receive a report that includes the agreements reached in the peer to peer call, a clinical summary, and recommendations for future use of medications."

# # #
Paladin Managed Care Services...
Paladin Managed Care Services
     http://www.paladinmc.com/

"Paladin Managed Care Services is setting the industry standard for services that reduce claims costs while improving patient care. Our unique approach combines physician-guided care with technology-driven efficiency to achieve better results for our clients, including insurance carriers, self-insured employers, insurance pools, municipalities, and group health organizations. In fact, we are the only managed care service provider that involves physicians in every service -- from case management and bill review to prescription approval and telephone support.

As an industry leader, Paladin is transforming managed care services and delivering extraordinary results through:
Physician-Guided Services: Physicians are involved in all our services -- Medical Bill Review, Case Management, Rx Utilization Management, Physician Guide, Utilization Review, and Comprehensive Claims Analysis."

# # #

Palladian Health http://www.palladianhealth.com/

Palladian Health   http://www.palladianhealth.com/
https://twitter.com/PalladianHealth

"Palladian Health was founded in Western New York almost twenty years ago as a chiropractic network and care management organization, working with major payers in the Northeastern U.S. to improve patient outcomes while reducing unnecessary medical expense.

Its range of service offerings evolved over the years to include Coordinated Spine Care in 2008, a proprietary process which improves the assessment and management of musculoskeletal pain from spinal disorders and promotes evidence-based decision making throughout the care cycle.

In 2015, Summer Street Capital, became the control owner of Palladian, putting a new leadership team into place. Palladian is now a leading NCQA-certified, URAC accredited musculoskeletal care management company focused on care management in orthopedics, physical therapy, chiropractic and related spine pain services partnering with payers across the United States.

Today, Palladian's broadened targeted customer base includes health insurers, TPAs, ACOs and large self-funded groups, focusing on the biomechanics, structure and function of the spine, its effects on the musculoskeletal system and synchronicity of these systems as they relate to the preservation and restoration of health."

# # #
Paramount Evaluation Group...
Paramount Evaluation Group
        http://paramountreview.com/
IME and file reviews

"Paramount Review Services is a national independent medical review company providing:

Independent Medical Examinations
Functional Capacity Evaluations
Peer/File Reviews
Bill Review
Case Management
Many other Independent Review Services

We have providers nationwide, and in every discipline, even many of the more unique. We offer examiners in every state; major cities as well as smaller towns.

Paramount services Insurance Claims Adjusters, Attorneys, Third Party Administrators, Employers and State Agencies with Auto, Workers' Compensation, Liability, and other Attorney requests."

# # #
Partners
Partners
        North Carolina
http://www.partnersbhm.org/
questions@partnersbhm.org

"You will often hear people call Partners a Managed Care Organization or MCO. Some call us a Local Management Entity-Managed Care Organization or LME-MCO. Both are true. Think of us as part government agency and part insurance company. All the money we manage is for serving the behavioral health care needs of you and others in your community. The better we manage that money, the more services and programs we can provide.

The North Carolina Department of Health and Human Services contracts with Partners to manage behavioral health care services paid with federal, state, and local taxes."

# # #
PDI

PDI
http://www.pdimcs.com/
hr@pdimcs.com

PDI maintains "all necessary licenses, permits, approvals and authorizations necessary in order to perform quality Disability Management Services in the Workers' Compensation Industry, which includes, Utilization/Peer Review, Nurse and Chiropractic Case Management and Maritime Case Management."

# # #
Peer Review Solutions...
Peer Review Solutions
http://www.peerreviewsolutions.com/
info@peerreviewsolutions.com

"Peer Review Solutions is a California-based, URAC-accredited independent review organization that provides objective, accurate and independent medical reviews of physicians and patient treatments to hospitals, insurance companies, attorneys, third party administrators, public agencies and large companies that retain our services. Our timely, cost-effective evaluations contribute to efficient case resolutions for our clients.

Physicians in our national network are licensed, credentialed, board-certified medical professionals with decades of experience across a broad range of specialties and subspecialties. These physicians have been carefully selected and trained for our network to ensure their adherence to strict medical and ethical standards. Our turnaround time for handling cases rigorously complies with URAC-specified requirements."

###
Peerlink Medical
Peerlink Medical
https://www.peerlinkmedical.com

# # #
PEI Healthcare Reviews
PEI Healthcare Reviews
http://peihealthcarereviews.com

# # #
Permedion
Permedion
http://hmspermedion.com/
https://twitter.com/HMSHealthcare

"Permedion, a wholly owned subsidiary of HMS, is a URAC-accredited, QIO-like entity. Permedion provides independent utilization and external medical review for both state government and private clients across the country to help ensure that inpatient and outpatient services are medically necessary, billed appropriately, and of the highest quality.

Our clients include Medicaid, state insurance departments, state medical boards, correctional departments, and other state agencies."

# # #
Physicians' Review Network http://www.prniro.com/
Physicians' Review Network
        http://www.prniro.com/
        recruiting@prniro.com

"PRN is an independent medical review organization providing expert, cost effective and unbiased reviews of healthcare services since 1995.

Our clients include all types of healthcare, disability, and workers compensation organizations..."

# # #
Physicians Review Organization...
Physicians Review Organization
        http://physiciansreview.org/
file reviews   padmin@physiciansreview.org

"Health care is one of our nation's most scrutinized industries. Facilities, medical staff, and insurers have an ever-increasing responsibility to maintain high-quality standards, provide transparency, and keep costs under control.

That's why a confidential and impartial external review is an essential tool for any health care facility or insurance provider. Whether the goal is improved quality of care, effective utilization of service, or provider review, a trusted review partner should be a critical part of your team."

"Physicians Review Organization provides case reviews to a wide range of partners including hospitals, physician practices, HMOs, managed care organizations, and major insurance companies."

# # #
PMA Companies http://www.pmacompanies.com/
PMA Companies   http://www.pmacompanies.com/
    https://twitter.com/pmacompanies

"PMA Companies provides risk management solutions and services in the U.S., specializing in workers' compensation, and offering property and casualty insurance. Headquartered in Blue Bell, PA, PMA has over a century of successful business experience.

PMA Companies is part of the Old Republic General Insurance Group, the largest business segment within Old Republic International (ORI)--one of the nation's 50 largest publicly held insurance organizations with a substantial interest in major segments of the industry. ORI is primarily a commercial lines underwriter, serving many of America's leading industrial and financial services companies as valued customers.

Since 1923, ORI has grown as a specialty insurance business, though its oldest subsidiary has insured lives since 1887. The organization's record as a long-term growth company is one of the best in the industry. Its performance reflects an entrepreneurial spirit, sound forward planning, and a corporate structure that promotes and encourages assumption of prudent business risks."

# # #
PMSCO Healthcare Consulting...
PMSCO Healthcare Consulting
        http://consultpmsco.com/

# # #
POMCO
POMCO
http://www.pomcogroup.com/
https://twitter.com/POMCOgroup

"One of the nation's largest third-party administrators offering fully customized solutions for benefits administration, risk management, and business process outsourcing needs."

# # #
Prest & Associates http://www.prestmds.com/
Prest & Associates http://www.prestmds.com/

file review (psych only)

"Prest & Associates, Inc. has more than two decades of experience providing
independent review in psychiatry, addiction medicine and behavioral healthcare."

# # #
Primaris
Primaris
http://primaris.org/
https://twitter.com/primaris_health
online@primaris.org

"Primaris is a healthcare consulting firm that works with hospitals, physicians and nursing homes to drive better health outcomes, improved patient experiences and reduced costs.

We take healthcare data and translate it into actionable quality improvement processes that create the foundation for highly reliable healthcare organizations.

Primaris has more than 30 years of experience advising healthcare organizations on how to improve quality, patient safety and clinical outcomes. In fact, as former physicians, nurses, and administrators, our consultants understand what it's like to be on the front line of healthcare."

# # #
PrimeWest
PrimeWest
www.primewest.org

"PrimeWest Health is a partnership of 13 rural Minnesota counties governed by a Joint Powers Board (JPB). Our JPB includes two county commissioners (one primary and one alternate) from each of our owner counties. We are headquartered in Alexandria, Minnesota. Since 1997 we have administered a County-Based Purchasing (CBP) health plan owned by the counties we serve. Through this health plan, we annually manage and pay for the health care, wellness, and human services of over 36,000 residents in our counties. What makes us different is our local county ownership structure and employees and the connection they have to the people we serve--because those people are our neighbors, family, or friends."

# # #
Principal
Principal
www.principal.com
https://twitter.com/Principal

"Whether you're a business, an institutional investor, or an individual preparing for the future, we can help you reach your goals through our best in class retirement services, insurance solutions, and asset management services.

Our offerings are based on experience--not quick wins or fads. Because we know that integrity, honesty, and comprehensive expertise are the right way to go--and the surest path to helping you reach your long-term financial stability goals."

# # #
Prium
Prium
http://www.prium.com/
IME, reviews

"Founded in 1987 as a utilization review company, PRIUM offers a complete portfolio of solutions that prevent and eliminate directionless workers' compensation claims. The hallmark of our offerings is the PRIUM Medical Intervention Program. This award-winning peer review program was developed to curb the increasing problem of prescription opioid fraud, misuse and abuse in workers' compensation.

By taking an evidence-based, relationship-focused approach that involves clinician-to-clinician discussions, PRIUM is more likely to obtain the agreement of treating physicians to modify the treatment plan. This, combined with PRIUM's effective oversight of implemented changes, has resulted in the elimination, weaning and reduction of thousands of inappropriate medications. Today this solution is considered the industry standard in closing the loop on complex claims.

We realize you have many options when it comes to a managed care and medical intervention services partner. But here's why our clients tell us that PRIUM is different:
Unmatched clinical expertise and jurisdictional experience that results in higher agreement rates and clinically-appropriate and compensable medical treatment
Exceptional operational efficiency that ensures on-time, accurate reviews thanks to our streamlined processes and proprietary tracking system called eCase

We get results. Our success comes from an outcomes focused approach driven by a companywide commitment to reducing unnecessary treatment
We turn bad claims into positive outcomes for the injured worker and you.

An Ameritox solutions provider, PRIUM sets the industry standard for workers' compensation medical interventions through its ability to secure higher agreement rates and to help ensure compliance with modified treatment plans. The hallmark of the medical intervention company's success is a collaborative physician engagement process encompassing evidence-based medicine, clinical oversight, and jurisdictional guidelines to facilitate optimal financial and clinical outcomes. PRIUM helps eliminate unnecessary treatment through a comprehensive approach that includes complex medical interventions, utilization reviews, urine drug monitoring, and independent medical exams."

###
Prizm
Prizm
www.prizmllc.com
https://twitter.com/PrizmLLC
IME and file reviews

"Prizm is a foremost provider of leading-edge technology and customer service to the medical management industry. Property and Casualty insurance providers rely on Prizm for the services they need to effectively manage personal injury protection (PIP) and medical liability, within an easy-to-use and environmentally-friendly work environment."

# # #
Procura Management
Procura Management

http://www.procura-inc.com/
proppo@procura-inc.com

"Our products and services enable better decisions and achieve better outcomes. They get injured people the right medications, products and services at the right time. They reduce program costs by looking beyond transactions, avoiding payments for medications and services that should not be paid, and pairing robust analytics with veteran clinical expertise. This leads to brighter insights and greater savings."

# # #
Professional Disability Associates (PDA)
Professional Disability Associates (PDA)
http://www.professionaldisabilityassociates.com/
pdareply@pdamaine.com
disability file reviews

"Professional Disability Associates is an innovative consulting company and an industry leader in providing specialty risk resources including medical and vocational consulting services to major disability insurers and self insured employers. PDA delivers customized solutions to our clients. We are trained and focused on the nuances of disability insurance. Our attention to quality is second to none.

PDA has the resources and ability to immediately provide broad levels of risk assessment ranging from claim related audits and peer reviews, to education and financial analysis to management consulting and coaching. PDA supports clients with a growing network of disability-trained physicians and nurses, covering over 35 specialties, master's level vocational consultants and many well respected insurance "veterans" in delivering specialized expertise and value to the industry.

This combination of strategic and operational resources delivers effective and efficient results to a client list that ranges from local small businesses to national and multinational corporations. We excel at delivering quality – the right level of expertise for the right level of business complexity and at the right cost."

# # #
Professional Evaluation Group
Professional Evaluation Group
http://pegime.com/
IME and file reviews
peg@pegime.com

"Professional Evaluation Group of Florida, Inc. (PEG) is a medical service group with a dedicated team specializing in the selection of board certified physicians and chiropractors who perform Independent Medical Evaluations (IMEs). We specialize in Personal Injury Protection (PIP), Liability, Workers Compensation, General Liability and Disability claims. We also do Record/Peer Reviews, Radiology Reviews and Bill Reviews.

We maintain a database in excess of 4000 board certified physicians and chiropractors nationwide with whom we schedule IMEs, Peer/Record Reviews and Film Reviews. The physicians we utilize are boarded in their specialties, licensed in their practicing states and have been verified by that state's court system.

PEG's physicians are available to review existing medical records, films, etc. and are familiar with the reporting requirements for the different casualty lines. All of our physicians are in private practice and are independent of PEG. The narrative reports that are completed and sent to our clients are dictated and signed by the physicians on their letterhead and are of the highest quality to meet the standards set forth by PEG.

Our goal is to help you make the most informed decision about the services you need. Our newly-designed 'Easy View Program' keeps you updated throughout the entire course of your file by viewing correspondences, appointment information and narrative reports. From beginning to end, we are confident you will be completely satisfied with your experience.

PEG has been servicing your needs since 1988. We believe our strength is our dedication to quality and our commitment to superior service."

# # #
Progeny Health
Progeny Health
http://www.progenyhealth.com/
        info@progenyhealth.com

"With passion and a singular focus, we improve the health outcomes of premature and medically complex newborns through provider collaboration and parental engagement."

# # #
ProPeer Resources
ProPeer Resources
http://www.propeer.com/
file reviews
(affiliated with Nexus MC)

"ProPeer Resources is your premier provider of independent specialty medical peer reviews. Since 1992, ProPeer Resources has been providing comprehensive and accurate independent medical peer reviews to claims departments across the nation - for health, disability, worker's compensation, auto/personal injury and life (accidental death) claims.

Recent customer satisfaction surveys have indicated that "Accuracy of Medical Peer Reviews" is what our clients value most in our services. Since its inception, ProPeer Resources' operational goals have included an initiative to provide our medical peer review process and services at speed and accuracy levels that exceed the competition. The company successfully attained that original goal by continually reducing the turn around time on Retrospective Medical Peer Reviews, and has now attained an average turn around time of less than three working days."

# # #
Provider Resources
Provider Resources
http://www.provider-resources.com/

"Provider Resources, Inc. (PRI) was established in 2003 with the mission to improve the nation's healthcare system and entered the federal sector in 2008. We are dedicated to supporting the healthcare community with compliance, integrity, and quality issues through education and efficient, innovative processes. We receive recognition for the application of problem-solving approaches for the healthcare industry due to the resources of our healthcare experts and corporate culture of compliance. The foundation of our success is based on standardized processes demonstrated by: URAC accreditation as an independent review organization (IRO)."

# # #
ProviDrs Care
ProviDrs Care
http://providrscare.net/

"ProviDRs Care is Kansas' only physician owned and managed PPO network in the state. Formerly known as WPPA and operational since 1985, ProviDRs Care works in partnership with insurance agents, brokers, insurance carriers, third party administrators, employers, health care providers and facilities to deliver cost-effective health services for Kansans.

ProviDRs Care enables there to be choice of health care plans by leasing its network to self-funded plans and insurance carriers. ProviDRs Care serves as the statewide PPO network for 15 nationally recognized carriers and 28 third party administrators.

Owned by the Medical Society of Sedgwick County, ProviDRs Care PPO network is built to deliver convenient access to complete healthcare services from physicians and hospitals that are highly respected in their communities. The network includes more than 11,000 practitioners, 157 hospitals and 700 outpatient facilities throughout Kansas as well as parts of Nebraska, Colorado and Missouri. By contracting with ProviDRs Care, these providers agree to perform healthcare services at a reduced fee.

Consumers with coverage accessing our network have lower out-of-pocket costs for healthcare services when they use a network provider."

# # #
Prudential
Prudential
www.prudential.com

"With operations in the United States, Asia, Europe and Latin America, we provide customers with a variety of products and services, including life insurance, annuities, retirement-related services, mutual funds and investment management. We strive to create long-term value for our stakeholders through strong business fundamentals, consistent with our mission guided by our vision and directed by our company's core values."

# # #
PsyBar

PsyBar
http://www.psybar.com/
IME and file reviews   (psych)

"PsyBar is one of the largest specialty providers of independent medical evaluations for employers and insurers. Services available include PsyBar's Fitness For Duty Assessments, Disability or Workers' Compensation Evaluations, and Risk Assessments. Risk managers, human resource directors, insurance claims managers and employee benefits professionals rely on PsyBar's network of 1,800 forensic professionals to ensure that their workforce is safe and productive."

# # #
PsychGroup
PsychGroup
http://psychgroup.com/

# # #
QDSI
QDSI
http://www.qdsi.com
IME and file reviews

"Qualified Disability Specialists, Inc. (QDSI) is regional network of recognized professionals who provide evidence-based medical opinions for a broad spectrum of Independent Medical Evaluation, Medical Record Reviews, Functional Capacity Evaluations, Disability, Veterans Exams and a host of other corporate medical related services. All QDSI services are expeditiously completed with the highest standards of professional credibility, accuracy and objectivity.

For over 20 years, QDSI has provided examinations and reporting excellence for, but not exclusive to, Third Party Administrators, Self-Insured Organizations, All Employees, Insurance Companies and Brokers, Disability Insurers and Managed Care Organization. Based on extensive research, QDSI also provides continuing professional support to attorneys, case managers and all our clients' needs."

# # #
QTC
QTC
www.qtcm.com
VA and other disability evals

"We Administer Examinations For:
Government/DoD programs; Third-party Administrators; Major Corporate Employers Private Insurance Companies"

# # #
Quad City Community Healthcare...

Quad City Community Healthcare
http://www.qcchealth.com/

"We specialize in meeting the needs of small employers and self insured employer groups. As a locally owned and operated health plan, QCCH is uniquely well suited to work with companies in the Quad Cities region in both Iowa and Illinois. At QCCH, our experience and industry knowledge allow us to create affordable solutions for your health insurance concerns. We provide competitively priced health insurance plans with hometown value through prompt and personal local service."

# # #
Qualis Health
Qualis Health
http://www.qualishealth.org/
https://twitter.com/qualishealth

"Qualis Health is one of the nation's leading population healthcare consulting organizations, partnering with our clients to improve care for millions of Americans every day. We work with public and private sector clients to advance the quality, efficiency and value of healthcare.

Qualis Health headquarters are in Seattle, Washington, with regional offices located in Alabama, Alaska, California, Idaho, the District of Columbia and New Mexico."

# # #

Quality Care Partners (QCP)...
Quality Care Partners (QCP)
http://www.qualitycarepartners.com/
info@qualitycarepartners.com

"Quality Care Partners (QCP) was initially developed as a local physician-hospital organization (PHO) incorporated in 1995. At the time QCP consisted of one hospital system and the local physicians from a 4 county area around Zanesville, Ohio. QCP has continued to evolve and change through the years. We pride ourselves on providing a complete range of healthcare benefit management services to help control cost and the premier network for Southeastern Ohio.

Throughout the years QCP has continued to grow and expand its business and in 2014, Quality Care Partners added 2 additional hospital systems to our board to become a Regional PHO. One of our many goals is to continue the growth of our board to include more hospital systems in our area."

# # #
Quality Medical Evaluations (QME)...
Quality Medical Evaluations (QME)
http://www.qmeval.com
IME and file reviews
info@QMEval.com

"Independent Medical Evaluations
Medical Record Peer Reviews
Medical Bill Audits/Repricing
Integrated Medical Peer Review

QME's professional team provides timely and defensible IMEs, Medical/Peer Reviews, and Medical Bill Repricing services. Our expert staff manages all aspects of our medical claim services with a focus on our 3 C's; Competency, Consistency and Communication."

# # #
Quality Review Services...
Quality Review Services
> http://www.qualityreviewservices.com/
> IME and file reviews
> qrs@qualityreviewservices.com

"QRS provides a full range of independent medical review services to insurers and the defense bar. Originally founded in 1994, QRS specializes in a full range of Independent Medical Examinations, Peer Reviews, Radiology Reviews, Diagnostic Reviews and Medical Record Retrieval. Our services are offered nationwide. We are available for liability, no fault, disability and worker?s compensation claims.

We understand that a thorough, accurate and expeditious medical evaluation clarifies many open issues of injury, causality and cost. This is crucial for effective claim analysis and determination."

# # #
Quantum Health
Quantum Health
http://quantum-health.com/

https://twitter.com/quantumhealth1

"For consultants who value more than the status quo, the Quantum Health model provides a distinct, proven alternative to the traditional ways currently used to help clients best contain healthcare costs. Our approach reorganizes an employer's benefits delivery model to bring together customer service, care management, and healthcare information under one roof. This allows us to engage more patients on a real-time basis and help them through their entire healthcare experience-- literally driving confusion and unnecessary costs out of the system.

Although the Quantum Health model garners interest, it's our results that really raise their eyebrows including:

First-year savings ranging from $134 to $976 per employee per year
3.9% CAGR over the first 3 years (net of all independent factors are accounted for and independently validated)
We have been successful in serving clients of various sizes in different industries and markets. Our "sweet spot" includes:

Self-funded employers across the United States
1,000 – 100,000 employees"

# # #
R3 Continuum
R3 Continuum

http://www.r3continuum.com
https://twitter.com/R3_Continuum

"R3 Continuum (R3) offers a continuum of solutions to assist organizations with every phase in the business planning, absence management, and return to work cycle. Collectively our services can ensure that organizations are ready for major disruptive events, able to respond successfully to these events (including workplace or threat of violence incidents), and equipped to accelerate employee recovery and return to work outcomes. R3 is a recognized leader in providing comprehensive solutions for complex claims and situations, and we guarantee to provide the right solutions with the right people at the right time.

We engage and partner with our clients using our expertise to solve their problems. We specialize in cases having a behavioral health component or comorbid diagnoses, responding to various levels of disruptive situations (e.g., mass layoffs, the death of an employee, or natural disasters), and varying degrees of workplace violence. In addition to our right solution, right people, right time, we guarantee to understand our client's business, to deliver creatively, and to create collaborative solutions."

They were kind enough to answer the survey questions:

• Is there a good contact person/department to give to physicians and/or psychologists in relation to recruitment/credentialing with your organization? Is there a desired contact method (ex: an email address or phone number) for them?

Yes, our network development group can be reached at network@r3continuum.com or via the form on our website at http://r3continuum.com/who-we-are/join-our-network/

• Do you contract directly with psychologists and/or neuropsychologists for medical records file review work or IME's?

Yes.

• Do you work directly with psychologists and/or physicians or do you go through third party companies? If so, which companies do you tend to use?

We work directly with our panelists.

• Do you contract directly w/ physicians for medical records file review work or IME's?

Yes.

• Do you ever have any employment opportunities for psychologists and/or neuropsychologists?

Yes.

• Do you ever have any employment opportunities for physicians?

Yes.

• If you employ psychologists and/or physicians, do you allow them to work from home?

Yes.

• Do you ever have any employment or contract opportunities for nurses in relation to file reviews and/or IME work?

Yes.

• Do you ever have any employment or contract opportunities for mental health counselors/social workers in relation to file reviews and/or IME work?

No, but we do contract and employ Master's-level mental health counselors and social workers in our disruptive event management practice. More information can be found at: http://r3continuum.com/workplace-resilience/

• Do any of your opportunities require the professional to be in active clinical practice and if so how do you define active clinical practice? (ex: how many hours per week? What percentage of income from direct treatment?)

Yes, we require our professionals to be in active clinical practice. Definitions vary by specialty.

• What opportunities, if any, do you have for professionals who are not currently in active clinical practice?

None.

• Do you contract/employ professionals nationwide or are there particular areas or regions of the country you work in; which areas of the country are you currently recruiting in?

We contract and employ professionals nationwide, needs vary by current customer load.

• Which physician specialties are you actively recruiting right now?

We are open to consideration for all specialties at this time.

• Are you actively seeking psychologists or neuropsychologists right now?

Yes.

• Can you provide estimates of a typical fee range that you tend to pay to psychologists and/or physicians for medical records file review and IME work (ex: do you have a typical hourly fee or per case fee/ per report fee that you are able to share)?

Sorry, pay rates for our panel are proprietary.

• Can you provide a brief company description that you'd like included in the book?

R3 Continuum believes people have a right to lead productive, meaningful lives. We help them do that with a suite of services that deal with potentially disruptive life events. Collectively, our services ensure that organizations are ready for major crisis events, able to respond successfully to these events (including workplace or threat of violence incidents), and equipped to accelerate employee recovery and return to work outcomes. R3 is a recognized leader in providing comprehensive solutions for complex claims and situations, and we guarantee to provide the right solutions with the right people at the right time. Visit our website at http://www.r3continuum.com

# # #
Read Reports, inc.
Read Reports, inc.
> https://www.read-reports.com/
> IME and file reviews

"All Medical Specialties; Services Nationwide"

"Independent Medical Examinations
Fit-for-Duty Evaluations
Police Exams (207-C)
Firefighter Exams (207-A)
Short & Long Term Disability

No Fault (Auto/PIP)
Bodily Injury
General Liability
Functional Capacity Evaluations
Peer Reviews
Records Reviews
Radiological Reviews
Transportation Services
Translation Services"

# # #
Reliable Clinical Experts (RCE)...
Reliable Clinical Experts (RCE)
> http://reliableclinicalexperts.com/
> Malpractice case reviews

# # #
Reliable Review Services...
Reliable Review Services
> http://www.ReliableRS.com
file reviews

"Reliable Review Services (RRS) is a URAC accredited Independent Peer Review Organization offering peer review and related medical review services to the Disability, Group Health, and Workers' Compensation markets."

# # #
Reliance Community Care Partners...
Reliance Community Care Partners
> http://relianceccp.org/

"Reliance Community Care Partners is a non-profit health care and case management organization that specializes in coordinating community health care services for older adults and those with disabilities.

Reliance is accredited by the Utilization Review Accreditation Council (URAC) for Case Management and Disease Management and employs Certified Case Managers (CCM)."

# # #
Review Med
Review Med
www.reviewmed.com
https://twitter.com/reviewmed
info@reviewmed.com

"Review Med is a national managed care firm that provides hands-on, personal communication and attention to customer needs. We have found that this approach ensures the best overall program for our clients while instilling confidence in our service and trust in our team.

Established as a corporation in 1997, Review Med provides Bill Review, Medical/Vocational Case Management and Return to Work Programs, Early Intervention Services, Medical Record Reviews, and Preauthorization/Pre-certification.

Since inception, our clinical expertise and team approach have been key to our foundation and growth. Combining this philosophy with the ever-changing technological advances, Review Med has emerged as a leader in the managed care industry providing quality services and high return on investment."

# # #
Richmond Disability Evaluation Group...
Richmond Disability Evaluation Group
> http://richmondevaluation.com/
> IME and file reviews
> NY, NJ, PA
> info@richmondevaluation.com

# # #
RisingMS
RisingMS
www.risingms.com
https://twitter.com/risingms

"Rising Medical Solutions offers a complete spectrum of solutions for
managing the costs and quality of medical care. Our integrated programs offer
the optimal care, at the appropriate time, for the right price."

They deliver "medical care and cost optimization solutions to the workers' comp, auto, liability and group health markets."

# # #

River Front Medical https://riverfrontpc.com/
River Front Medical   https://riverfrontpc.com/
IME

"Occupational Health Services
Health & Wellness Programs
Drug & Alcohol Testing & Administration
Independent Medical Evaluations"

# # #
RKI Claims Specialists https://rkiclaims.com
RKI Claims Specialists   https://rkiclaims.com
          IME and file reviews

"The physicians on our national panel are all board
certified, licensed professionals in their field. We
consistently review our panel to make sure all
physicians maintain the highest standards of quality
and meet our credentialing guidelines. Our physicians
understand the importance of providing our customers
with a high quality IME!"

# # #
Sandhills Center
Sandhills Center
          North Carolina
          http://www.sandhillscenter.org/

"Sandhills Center manages public mental health,
intellectual/developmental disabilities and substance
use disorder services for the citizens of Anson,
Guilford, Harnett, Hoke, Lee, Montgomery, Moore,
Randolph and Richmond counties.

As a publicly-funded Local Management Entity-Managed Care Organization (LME-MCO), Sandhills Center does not provide services directly, but acts as an agent of the North Carolina Department of Health & Human Services. Sandhills Center ensures that citizens in our region who seek services are able to access them through a network of contracted private providers.

We partner with individuals, family members, service providers, policy makers and other community stakeholders in creating, managing and supporting quality behavioral health services that meet the needs of our communities."

# # #
Scion Dental
Scion Dental
        Dental claims management
http://www.sciondental.com

# # #
Scope Medical
Scope Medical
http://www.imeexams.com/
IME and file reviews

"Independent Medical Examinations (IMEs)
Record Reviews (RORs)
Pre-Employment Psychological Screenings (Police, Fire, Public Servants)
Peer Reviews
Plaintiff Experts

Diagnostic Reviews
Durable Medical Equipment Reviews
Bill Audits
Disability Examinations (Long Term & Short Term)
Functional Capacity Evaluations (FCEs)
Fitness for Duty Evaluations (FMLA)
Psychiatric Profiles
Legal Appearances (Depositions, Court, Arbitrations)
Claims Defense"

"Physicians - Earn extra money doing IMEs and
Reviews

Earn an additional $5,000 to $75,000 per year--you
decide how much you want to work
Work can be done at office locations in Stoneham,
Dorchester, Brockton, Fall River, Taunton,
Yarmouthport, Worcester, and Springfield--or in your
own private office
Hours are available on Saturdays and early evenings as
well as the rest of the business week
Specialties Needed: Board certified Orthopedic
Surgeons, Chiropractors, Physical Therapists, and
Specialists in Neurology/Surgery, Cardiology, Internal
Medicine, ENT, OB-GYN, Hand Surgery, Psychiatry,
and others

How It Works

Scope Medical is a provider of Independent Medical Exams and Medical Record Reviews. We hire a network of physicians and market their services to our clients, insurance companies. We typically book a physician's time 6-8 weeks out and have them go to one of our facilities for a set period of time (i.e. 4-7pm in our Stoneham office). We would schedule 6-10 patients during that period of time.

The physician interviews each patient, reviews any medical records that are available and performs a physical examination. They then release the patient and dictate their findings to a toll free dictation service. We provide a format to follow and each case will have specific questions to be answered. When the transcription is completed (usually 24 hours) we email the report to the physician for review and electronic signature. Periodically we need physicians to simply review records and dictate a report following a format we provide.

About Scope Medical
Founded in 2001, Scope Medical has successfully completed over twenty thousand IMEs and reviews for over 200 clients. We have over 500 physicians on staff and add more each month. We are headquartered in Stoneham, Massachusetts, with 15 additional exam locations throughout New England. Scope founders Kathy D'Amore and Katherine Jordan have over 25 years combined experience in the independent medical exam industry. Their personal touch and involvement building relationships with clients and physicians keeps Scope Medical one of the top IME providers."

# # #
SDA (Southern Diagnostic Associates)...
SDA (Southern Diagnostic Associates)
>   https://www.sdaime.com/services.htm
>   IME and file reviews

"SDA's medical review services include Independent
Medical Exams (IMEs), Peer Reviews, Disability Exams,
Record and Utilization Reviews, MRI and X-Ray
Reviews and Diagnostic Interpretations in all
specialties along with evaluation programs for Group
Health, Workers' Compensation as well as Disability
Claims and Auto / General Liability Insurance carriers,
Third-Party Administrators and Law Firms,
Governmental Agencies, Health Insurers and Benefits
Administrators.

We will make onsite visits and copy medical records,
whenever possible schedule the same day with an
appropriately licensed physician, manage all
preparatory work and provide a comprehensive,
definitive and timely final report. We handle the
scheduling of appointments and notification of the
parties, transportation if needed, an interpreter when
required plus all follow-ups related to our services.

SDA takes pride in our best practices for delivering the
highest quality medical review services. Preferred
providers will determine an accurate, current diagnosis
and make recommendations for ongoing treatment. In
addition, we will address any other issues relevant to
the case, such as causality, reasonableness of care or
medical necessity."

"Types of Reviews

Independent Medical Reviews – A process where expert independent medical professionals are selected to determine causal relationship, medical status and the appropriateness of the current medical treatment plan, etc. SDA requires all reports to be independently processed by the medical provider, typed and forwarded on their own stationary. SDA does not participate in the production of the reports, ensuring an arms length transaction for our clients. SDA reviews all reports to ensure that essential components of the report are present and that your questions are answered. The medical opinions rendered are those of the examining physician and based upon his/her clinical assessment and review of medical records. Also an objective medical assessment of your claimant to assist you in determining claim compensability and/or liability, restrictions and limitations, employability or disability status. The evaluation is deemed "independent" because the physician who conducts the evaluation is a private practitioner who is neither the examinee's treating physician nor an employee of the client who requests the evaluation. SDA will provide an IME conducted by one or more physicians, depending on your needs. We can even coordinate a panel evaluation for you if you have a complex case requiring the perspectives of different specialties.

Peer Reviews - A Medical Peer Review is a process whereby providers evaluate the quality of work performed by their colleagues, in order to determine compliance with accepted health care standards. This review is generally a retrospective consideration by a medical professional of equal standard.

Utilization Reviews - A Utilization Review is a review performed to determine the necessary, appropriate, and efficient allocation of health care resources and services given or proposed to be given to a patient. Review may be conducted concurrently or retrospectively. This process uses objective clinical criteria to ensure the services are medically necessary and provided at the appropriate level of care.

Workers' Compensation – Utilization and Peer Reviews - The reasonableness or necessity of all treatment provided by a health care provider under the Workers' Compensations act may be subject to prospective, concurrent or retrospective utilization review at the request of an employee, employer, or insurer. It is a review of pertinent bills to determine medical necessity and appropriateness of treatment.

Workers' Compensation – IMEs - Independent Medical Examinations are evaluations performed by an evaluator not involved in the care of the examinee, for clarifying clinical and case issues. IMEs are an important component of workers' compensation systems, and are also used to clarify other disability or liability associated cases. Impairment evaluations are often used to provide a more objective understanding of the impact of an injury or illness. The quality of examinations and examiners varies widely, however, having been in the business for more than 25 years, SDA has successfully identified skilled, thorough and unbiased examiners.

Film Reviews – A review of the actual MRI's, CT scans, or X-ray images read by a board certified radiologist to determine the diagnostic impression"

# # #
SEAK
SEAK
www.SEAK.com
advertising directories/training conferences (they don't actually provide referrals, but you may be interested in advertising in their directory)

Are SEAK's directories worth the money? In the Summer of 2016 I conducted a survey of over 500 physicians and psychologists who were listed in SEAK's file review directory; 163 responded. Of those who responded, 50.31% (82 people) reported that over the past year they had received zero referrals because of their listing in the directory. I personally received two over the course of a little more than one year on the directory. I didn't conduct a survey for the IME directory or any of the other directories out there from SEAK or other companies. You can see the full results of the file review-related survey at: http://www.reviewsandIMEs.com/data.pdf

# # #
Secure Health
Secure Health
http://www.shpg.com/

"Secure Health is a third party administrator (TPA) and preferred provider organization (PPO) network located in Macon, Georgia. We are owned by physician-hospital organizations and have managed health benefits for employers with self-funded health benefit plans since 1992. Today, we serve over 72 health plans in multiple states across the U.S.

Our primary goal is to minimize costs while providing excellent service for our members. Our services are designed to help members become healthy and stay healthy. Each plan is tailored to its unique population, and our results illustrate greater coordinated medical care, member satisfaction, and lower overall plan costs."

# # #
Sedgwick
Sedgwick
http://www.sedgwick.com
        https://twitter.com/Sedgwick

"Sedgwick Claims Management Services, Inc., is a leading global provider of technology-enabled risk and benefits solutions. At Sedgwick, caring countsSM; the company takes care of people and organizations by delivering cost-effective claims, productivity, managed care, risk consulting and other services through the dedication and expertise of more than 14,000 colleagues in some 275 offices located in the U.S., Canada, the U.K and Ireland. Sedgwick facilitates financial and personal health and helps customers and consumers navigate complexity by designing and implementing customized programs based on proven practices and advanced technology that exceed expectations."

# # #
Sheakley
Sheakley
http://www.sheakley.com/
https://twitter.com/sheakley1

"Sheakley is a family owned, outsourced human resources specialty firm dedicated to recognizing and meeting the growing needs of employers. We offer tailored solutions that help our clients attract, care for, protect, manage, and reward their most valuable asset/their employees.

Serving employers since 1963, we've evolved beyond our industry leading workers' comp and unemployment claims management, to now consistently and expertly offer and service comprehensive HR solutions. We proudly represent more than 50,000 clients. As a nationally recognized leader in the human resources and employee benefits industry, we provide our clients the freedom to focus on their core business. Having engaged Sheakley, they more than simply consider it done. They know, trust and value that it's done right."

# # #
Signet Claim Solutions
Signet Claim Solutions
http://www.signetcs.com
IME and file reviews   getinfo@signetcs.com

"Signet Claim Solutions, LLC offers the insurance industry the tools needed to help manage the claims evaluation process.

• Independent Medical Examinations
• Peer (File) Reviews
• Radiology Reviews

- Legal Nurse Review (LNC)
- Medical Coding Review
- Medical Records Retrieval"

# # #
SIHO
SIHO
http://www.siho.org/

"SIHO Insurance Services was founded in 1987 by local employers, hospitals and physicians to provide a solution to rising health care costs for local businesses. SIHO is now a dominant employee health care benefits company, providing health plans to any size business.

SIHO Headquarters
As a comprehensive health care organization, SIHO Insurance Services provides any type of health plan a business may desire. On the leading edge of employee health benefits, SIHO provides claims administration, pre-certification, case management, concurrent review, utilization review, member services, benefit consulting, a national pharmacy network and a comprehensive network of hospitals and physicians in one facility.

SIHO's Vision/Mission/Values

Integrated Delivery System

SIHO Insurance Services provides integrated delivery of quality health care through a system local to our communities and unified in its operations and technology. SIHO Insurance Services was created nearly two decades ago as a collaborative and cooperative effort of community parties which have an interest in the quality and efficiency of health care delivery: the hospitals, physicians, employers and citizens.

These functions include the following:
Medical Management
Chronic Disease Management
Managed Pharmacy Program
Network Services
Plan Features
Account Management
Client Services
Employer Benefits

SIHO Insurance Services' success in providing quality health care to employees at an affordable cost to employers has resulted in continuous growth."

# # #
Social Security Disability
Social Security Disability
Consultative Evaluations (an IME) or in-house file review (but usually you are not able to be a provider for both services at the same time).

While there are other options such as disability hearings/the office of adjudication and review, and regional offices performing quality reviews, the best place to start out is by contacting a PRO at the DDS (disability determination service) that is closest to you; here is a state by state directory of PRO's on SSA's website:
https://ssa.gov/disability/professionals/procontacts.htm

Social Security is not known for being one of the more lucrative sources for file review or examinations, however they make up for it by being consistent. There are lots of applicants out there and typically there is plenty of work. If you are interested in file review with a DDS you are unlikely to be able to do this work from home however. You'd probably have to do this from the location of one of the state DDS offices.

# # #
Solstice Benefits...
Solstice Benefits   http://www.solsticebenefits.com/
        https://twitter.com/solsticedental

"Dental, vision and life benefits plans to groups and consumers."

# # #
South Florida Utilization Review...
South Florida Utilization Review
        http://www.sfur.com/
file reviews

"We specialize in Workers Compensation Claims Review, Bill Negotiation and Insurance Peer Review, applying medical knowledge and financial best practices to benefit our customers."

"It's been our privilege supporting customers across the US for over 30 years. We continually strive to improve and innovate our services to best meet our customers' ongoing challenges."

###
Southern Diagnostic Associates
Southern Diagnostic Associates
https://www.sdaime.com
"SDA is the oldest medical claims consulting firm in Florida. We are now in our 26th year striving each and every day to exceed our clients' expectations by providing a wide array of services to create efficiencies in managing and assessing the validity of medical claims and cases. This is accomplished by bringing together a medical staff of experienced, board-certified experts who are recognized experts in their field and have demonstrated an understanding of complex medico-legal issues. The team at SDA functions in an environment in which they are given full support of a dedicated administrative staff knowledgeable in both medicine and law with the surroundings of a pleasant, modern facility."

# # #
Specialty Benefits Services...
Specialty Benefits Services
        http://specialtybenefitservices.com/

"Express Scripts Specialty Benefit Services is our revolutionary approach to enhancing patient care and solving plan sponsors' specialty cost challenges. We provide the most comprehensive range of specialty management and utilization services -- across both the medical and pharmacy benefit."

# # #
Spooner Medical Administrators...
Spooner Medical Administrators
>   http://www.medadmin.com/
>   Ohio; workers comp MCO

# # #
Standard
Standard
www.standard.com
insurance company

"StanCorp Financial Group, Inc., and its primary subsidiaries: Standard Insurance Company, The Standard Life Insurance Company of New York, StanCorp Investment Advisers, Inc., Standard Retirement Services, Inc. and StanCorp Mortgage Investors, LLC."

# # #
Statewide IME Services
Statewide IME Services
http://statewideime.com/
IME
info@statewideime.com

"Statewide IME Services LLC offers independent medical evaluations in the New York Tri-state region and nationwide   "

# # #
Strategic Claims Solutions...
Strategic Claims Solutions
> http://www.strategicclaimssolutions.com

"We are a resource for insurance claim cost containment that specializes in second injury recovery, medical record retrieval, Prescription Drug Reviews and claim consulting services.
Our mission is to help our clients reach their cost containment goals by providing cost effective services that will save both time and money.
We put our claim expertise to work for our clients in the following areas:
Medical Records Canvass
Medical Records Retrieval
Medical Records Review and Summary
Prescription Drug Reviews"

# # #
Stubbe & Associates
Stubbe & Associates
http://www.stubbe.com/
> Info@stubbe.com

"Stubbe & Associates is a National Medical and Vocational Case Management firm dedicated to providing the highest level of service in the most cost-effective manner possible. We have unmatched coverage in the Regional Midwestern states where the company was first established in 1986. With solid growth, Stubbe & Associates has added offices, staff and a network of coverage throughout the United States.

We answer our phones and respond to emails, faxes and online referrals 7am – 7pm (central time zone); effectively supporting our clientele on both the East and West Coasts. If you are looking for case management that will meticulously attend to the complicated issues associated with your file then look no further. The dedicated, enthusiastic and accomplished professionals of Stubbe & Associates' are what you have found.

We are committed to...

Assisting our clients in achieving the highest possible level of function
Our customers, who are so valuable to us that we must consistently exceed their expectations
Communicating and reporting all information in a timely manner
Honesty, integrity and professionalism in our work
Success as a team and as an organization"

# # #
Sun Life

Sun Life
http://www.sunlife.com/
https://twitter.com/sunlife

"Sun Life Financial is a leading provider of employee benefits in the U.S. Our mission? To help people protect what they love about their lives."

# # #
Superior Medical Consultants
Superior Medical Consultants
        http://smcexams.com/
IME
info@smcexams.com

"Providing Independent Medical Evaluations for insurance companies, third party administrators, self-insured employers, and the legal community."

"We provide IME's throughout New York State (including the 5 Burroughs of New York City) and Nationally."

# # #
Support Claim Services...
Support Claim Services
        www.supportclaimservices.com
IME and file reviews

"SCS provides efficient medical cost containment services with quality evaluations and professional services. Utilizing advanced technology, the Company processes No-Fault, Liability and Workers Compensation Claims and also offers a national Bill Review Program all through its virtual claims system."

# # #
Symetra
Symetra
www.symetra.com
https://twitter.com/symetra

"Symetra Life Insurance Company is a subsidiary of Symetra Financial Corporation, a diversified financial services company based in Bellevue, Washington. In business since 1957, Symetra provides employee benefits, annuities and life insurance through a national network of benefit consultants, financial institutions, and independent agents and advisors."

# # #
Telligen
Telligen
http://www.telligen.com/
https://twitter.com/telligen

"Do you deliver healthcare? Or pay for healthcare? No matter your role, Telligen can help you improve quality and lower costs by combining our deep clinical and technical expertise to solve your healthcare challenges. We are passionate about turning raw data into knowledge and knowledge into action. It's what we call "Healthcare Intelligence."

# # #
The Coordinating Center...
The Coordinating Center
> www.coordinatingcenter.org
> https://twitter.com/CoordinatingCen

"The mission of The Coordinating Center is to partner with people of all ages and abilities and those who support them in the community to achieve their aspirations for independence, health and meaningful community life."

# # #
The Hanover Insurance Group...
The Hanover Insurance Group
> http://www.hanover.com/
> https://twitter.com/The_Hanover

"The Hanover Insurance Group, Inc., based in Worcester, Mass., is the holding company for several property and casualty insurance companies, which together constitute one of the largest insurance businesses in the United States. For more than 160 years, The Hanover has provided a wide range of property and casualty products and services to individuals, families, and businesses. The Hanover distributes its products through a select group of independent agents and brokers. Together with its agents, the company offers specialized coverages for small and mid-sized businesses, as well as insurance protection for homes, automobiles, and other personal items. Through its international member company, Chaucer, The Hanover also underwrites business at Lloyd's of London in several major insurance and reinsurance classes, including marine, property and energy."

# # #
The Hartford
The Hartford
www.thehartford.com
https://twitter.com/TheHartford

"As a company in business for more than 200 years, we understand what it means to be sustainable. We have helped people and businesses prepare for the unexpected, protect what is uniquely important to them, and prevail through life's challenges and opportunities. We do this by delivering industry leading property and casualty insurance, group benefits and mutual funds to our customers, creating a diverse and inclusive culture for our employees, financial performance for our shareholders, and by engaging with and serving the communities in which we work and live."

# # #
The Health Plan
The Health Plan
www.healthplan.org
https://twitter.com/TheHealthPlanHQ

"We are The Health Plan – known for exceptional personal service and delivering clinically-driven, technology-enhanced, customer-focused insurance products and services that manage and improve the health and well-being of our members."

# # #
The Physician Network
The Physician Network
        https://tpnexpert.com/
        https://twitter.com/tpnexpert
IME and file reviews

"The Physician Network (TPN) provides expert medical review and examination services to the insurance, legal and private industries throughout the USA."

# # #
The Prime Network
The Prime Network
www.theprimenetwork.com

IME and file reviews   info@theprimenetwork.com

"THE PRIME NETWORK is a national and regional provider of Peer Reviews (PRO), Independent/Defense Medical Evaluations (IME/DME), and other related services by Board Certified Providers to insurance companies, employers, attorneys, case management professionals and others. Our primary goal is to provide fast report turnaround times while delivering objective, clear and concise reports."

# # #
TMF
TMF
www.tmf.org

"TMF Health Quality Institute focuses on promoting quality health care through contracts with federal, state and local governments, as well as private organizations. For more than 40 years, TMF has helped health care providers and practitioners in a variety of settings improve care for their patients.

TMF was chartered in 1971 as a private, nonprofit organization of licensed physicians (MDs and DOs) to lead quality improvement and medical review efforts in Texas. Originally known as the Texas Medical Foundation, the company changed its name to TMF Health Quality Institute in 2005 to reflect the expansion of its work throughout the nation.

Since 1984, TMF has been the Centers for Medicare & Medicaid Services' Quality Improvement Organization (QIO) for Texas, improving care provided to Medicare beneficiaries through cooperative efforts with the health care community. In 2014, TMF became the Quality Innovation Network QIO for a region comprising Texas, Arkansas, Missouri, Oklahoma and Puerto Rico, improving cardiac health, reducing disparities in diabetes care, improving prevention efforts through meaningful use of health information technology, reducing infections in hospitals, reducing harm in nursing homes, assisting providers with quality reporting and helping communities improve the coordination of health care for patients to reduce unnecessary hospital readmissions and adverse drug events.

TMF's expansive reach in health care continues with the Comprehensive Primary Care initiative through the Center for Medicare & Medicaid Innovation. The initiative seeks to improve care, improve health and lower costs for patients and their families in the primary care setting. This is accomplished through enhanced care coordination, care management and health information technology.

Through this project, TMF works with approximately 500 physician practices, serving about 385,000 Medicare and Medicaid beneficiaries, in seven U.S. regions. TMF is the lead contractor overseeing the project's National Learning Network – a mix of Web-based and live, face-to-face events, with a curriculum for participating practices as well as learning opportunities through peer brainstorming and sharing of best practices for collective problem solving.

In 2011, TMF acquired C2C Solutions, Inc., a Medicare Qualified Independent Contractor with offices in Florida and employees throughout the nation. This acquisition expanded TMF's scope of services and increased our presence in the government contracting market. C2C specializes in providing health care sector support and administrative services in the handling of Medicare second-level appeals. It adjudicates second-level Medicare Part A appeals from 24 western states and three U.S. territories. In addition, C2C adjudicates second-level Medicare Part B appeals for the entire U.S. and its territories. The Medicare Part A West task order and the Medicare Part B South task order, which added 15 states and two territories, thereby completing Medicare Part B coverage of the entire U.S., were awarded to C2C in 2014. The company also conducts reconsiderations of initial Medicare claim determinations concerning durable medical equipment (DME) across the entire U.S. and its territories. C2C has processed more than 4.1 million QIC claims adjudications.

In 2013, TMF established the TMF Foundation in support of TMF's vision to improve lives by improving the quality of health care. The TMF Foundation provides resources and educational support to organizations focused on the health of Texas residents. Recently, the foundation joined an effort to affect the trend of childhood obesity. In partnership with the Texas PTA, the foundation is championing an initiative that finds and rewards children making healthy eating choices in the K-5 school lunchroom. A second new project is one in which children age 3-5 are motivated and taught about physical activity, health, gardening and healthy eating behaviors.

The foundation also continues teaching people with diabetes how to control and monitor their disease through the successful ¡Adelante! program, which began in 2013 to provide education and resources at no cost to populations at high risk for diabetes.

We partner with health care providers in multiple settings:

Hospitals
Physician Offices
Nursing Homes
Home Health Agencies
Medication Safety and Reduction of Adverse Drug Events
TMF partners with health care providers to ensure that every patient receives the right care... every time."

# # #

Trillium Health Resources...
Trillium Health Resources
> http://www.trilliumhealthresources.org/

"Trillium Health Resources is a local governmental agency (LME/MCO) that manages mental health, substance use and intellectual/developmental disability services in a 24-county area in eastern North Carolina. Our responsibility is to connect individuals and families to the help they need when they need it. We are responsible for managing state and federally funded services for people who receive Medicaid, are uninsured or cannot afford services."

# # #
Tristar Managed Care...
Tristar Managed Care
> http://www.tristarmanagedcare.com/

"TRISTAR Managed Care has 17 years of experience providing Bill Review, offering access to PPO Network contracts as well as nationwide Medical Provider Networks (MPN) for self-insured and insured organizations.

TMC analyzes and reduces medical bills to fair and equitable amounts. Statistics show that over half of the costs of a Workers' Compensation claim are for medical benefits. TMC closely monitors medical treatment plans and bills in order to reduce workers' compensation costs. We average savings of more than 70% for all types of medical bills. TMC's highly trained analysts review all unidentified and complex procedures prior to processing. By reading the medical reports, TMC ensures that the services billed were the services rendered. Our trained, experienced analysts add up to 30% additional savings to the bill review engine. We recruit the best analysts in the industry, each averaging 15 years of experience. All of our analysts undergo intensive training which includes testing, lecture, and actual hands on practice, with continual monitoring by supervisors throughout the duration of their employment."

# # #
UMC Medical
UMC Medical
www.umc4ime.com
IME
physician-recruiting@umc4ime.com

"UMC Medical Consultants, P.C. is a URAC-accredited, physician-owned and operated company specializing in Independent Medical Evaluations and related health services throughout New York State and the whole country."

# # #

UniMex
UniMex
www.umepc.com
IME
exams@umepc.com

"UniMex is an organization of service oriented, caring employees, with over 35 years of collective experience, who have networked thousands of Doctors, worldwide, to provide the highest quality independent medical examinations available today."

# # #
UnitedHealthcare
UnitedHealthcare
www.uhc.com
https://twitter.com/myUHC

"UnitedHealthcare is an operating division of UnitedHealth Group, the largest single health carrier in the United States."

# # #
United Review Services
United Review Services
https://www.unitedreview.com

# # #
University Disability Consortium
University Disability Consortium
http://www.universitydisabilityconsortium.com/
primarily file reviews
info@universitydisabilityconsortium.com
udc@udc1.com

"University Disability Consortium is a Boston-based, physician owned and managed multi-disciplinary network of ABMS board-certified physicians, psychologists, neuropsychologists, nurses, and vocational rehabilitation professionals specializing in the performance of fair and unbiased medical file reviews, panel reviews, independent medical evaluations (IMEs), panel IMEs, and expert witness testimony. We are also well regarded for our expertise in working with attorneys in forensic medical screenings."

# # #
Unum
Unum
www.unum.com
https://twitter.com/unumnews

"Unum's four distinct , but similarly focused businesses – Unum US, Unum UK, Colonial Life, and Starmount Life – are each a market leader in making disability, life, accident, critical illness, dental and vision insurance accessible in the workplace.

Our customers know they can count on Unum when the unexpected occurs. 33 million people at 181,000 companies rely on Unum's products and services – including a third of Fortune 500 companies – and we paid out more than $6.8 billion in benefits last year to individuals and families who were impacted by life-changing events."

# # #
USAble life
USAble life
www.usablelife.com

"USAble Life is an insurance provider in 49 states (excluding NY) and the District of Columbia. We are part of the holding company, Life & Specialty Ventures, and uniquely owned by multiple BlueCross BlueShield plans. We also offer our products through many non-owner Blue plans across the US.

We work with brokers, business owners, schools and other organizations to bring benefits to employees. Focusing on the "other side" of benefits, those beyond health insurance – life, disability, dental, vision, accident plans, critical illness and cancer, hospital confinement and more, our products and services protect the financial well-being of individuals by providing cash during their time of need.

Our benefit offering consists of more than 20 products and services and we are continually expanding these offerings to create new solutions to financial challenges and life in general. Our solutions help organizations provide value to employees while maintaining a bottom line focus. Simply put, we provide peace of mind."

# # #
Utopia Claims Concepts...
Utopia Claims Concepts
http://www.utopiaclaims.com/

IME and file reviews   info@utopiaclaims.com

"Utopia Claims Concepts, Inc. provides quality Independent Medical Evaluations (IMEs), Radiological Reviews and Peer Reviews in all medical fields. We specialize in Workers' Compensation, No Fault & Bodily Injury Claims. We are authorized by The New York State Workers' Compensation Board to conduct IMEs and all of our physicians are Board Certified"

# # #
Vaya Health (formerly Smoky Mountain MCO)
Vaya Health (formerly Smoky Mountain MCO)
     North Carolina
     www.vayahealth.com

"Vaya Health is a public managed care organization (MCO) that oversees Medicaid, federal, state and local funding for services and supports related to mental health, substance use and intellectual/ developmental disability (IDD) needs. We operate in 23 western North Carolina counties that are home to over 1 million residents who may be eligible for our prevention, treatment and crisis services."

###
Veterans' Attorneys
Veterans' Attorneys

If you understand the VA's disability system you can offer independent medical opinion file reviews (and/or exams) on veteran's disability claims (ex: writing things like Nexus letters). You would perform this work for the veteran/veteran's attorney themselves.

# # #
Veteran Compensation and Pension Medical...
Veteran Compensation and Pension Medical Consulting Services
www.vetcompandpen.com
VA disability evals

# # #
Veterans Evaluation Services (VES)...
Veterans Evaluation Services (VES)
    www.vesservices.com
    (877)637-8387
VA disability evals

# # #
Vocational Rehabilitation
Vocational Rehabilitation
The specific agencies involved vary by state.

# # #
Voya Financial
Voya Financial
www.voya.com
https://twitter.com/Voya

"Voya Financial, Inc. (NYSE: VOYA), helps Americans plan, invest and protect their savings -- to get ready to retire better. With a clear mission to make a secure financial future possible -- one person, one family, one institution at a time -- Voya's vision is to be America's Retirement Company™."

# # #
WellComp
WellComp
https://www.wellcomp.com/

"WellComp has been a leading national provider of managed care services. We've specialized in Workers' Compensation cost containment since 1985, and our team has the experience and expertise to create and manage custom solutions that deliver cost savings to clients and the appropriate care to injured workers. Our processes are URAC accredited and many of our 350 employees are certified specialists in their areas.

Our services include:

Case Management
Utilization Review
Medical Bill Review
National and Specialty Proprietary PPO Networks
National Diagnostic Imaging And Scheduling Network
Nurse Triage
Pharmacy Benefit Management
Medicare Secondary Payer Compliance Services

Our services offerings are available on a stand-alone or integrated basis so we can create custom solutions that meet each client's specific needs and factor in their specific medical and cost management guidelines."

###
Wellpoint
Wellpoint
Canada
http://wellpointhealth.ca

# # #
Windham Group
Windham Group
> http://www.windhamgroup.com/
> Managed care, IME and file reviews

"Windham Group began in 1989 and resides in New Hampshire's Merrimack Valley, a place with a unique history in work environment ethics. Ever since the industrial revolution, the plight of the working person has become a central pillar in our country, and we are reminded daily of these issues by our mill yard surroundings. We see the history of our working nation and of our local area as the history of Return to Work, and find purpose in remembering where we've come from.

This is where we work! The Amoskeag mill yard was once the largest cotton textile plant in the world, powered by the mighty Merrimack River. This place was pivotal in redefining human productivity during the industrial revolution. America would not be what it is today without this powerful era, and yet, so many were strained beyond capacity in order to remain employed on small sums of money.

Many of these mills along the Merrimack until recently, lay abandoned. Our mill is almost as alive and buzzing as it was 150 years ago, however, instead of weaving fabrics and working machines, we are weaving work solutions and working to keep folks productive at their regular job post injury.

We believe that our city, nation, and world, are entering a new era where an attention to work environment sustainability will become increasingly important as technology advances and the role of human ergonomics is brought to the forefront. Our commitment to addressing injury and recovery issues at their core is driven by a heightened awareness of these trends of development and the new measures that will be required in thinking more deeply than our competitors about Return to Work."

# # #
Workers Compensation
Workers Compensation
(varies by state; aka Workman's   Compensation).
Here is a website with links to state workers' compensation programs:

http://www.genexservices.com/news-insights/state-workers-compensation-agencies

We generally think of the state programs which vary from state to state. However, you may also be interested in a federal program (Division of Federal Employees' Compensation). "The Federal Employees' Compensation Act provides workers' compensation coverage to three million federal and postal workers around the world for employment-related injuries and occupational diseases. The Division of Federal Employees' Compensation (DFEC) has responsibility for administering the Act through its twelve district offices and national office."
Learn more here:
https://www.dol.gov/OWCP/DFEC/

# # #
Workplace Health Solutions http://www.whsny.com/
Workplace Health Solutions
        http://www.whsny.com/
IME (NY)

"Workplace Health Solutions is a preferred source for employers to access networks of providers in New York State. We are committed to our network of providers who are top notch and are part of our service delivery to support employers in their desire to increase productivity and return healthy employees to the workplace.

Our primary goal is to partner with providers who will commit to timely appointments, objective feedback on diagnosis, and offer treatment recommendations that will return the injured worker to the workplace as quickly as medically appropriate"

# # #
WVMI
WVMI
http://www.wvmi.org/

"WVMI is a not-for-profit company focused on measuring and improving health care quality. We are headquartered in Charleston, WV with offices in Virginia, Pennsylvania, Delaware and New Jersey. We are a group of more than 200 physicians, nurses, health services researchers, statisticians, data analysts and educators dedicated to "improving the people we serve." We are actively working to help achieve the National Quality Strategy and its three goals of better care, smarter spending and healthier people. We strive to be a change agent, trusted partner and integrator of local organizations collaborating to improve care."

51297796R00161

Made in the USA
Middletown, DE
01 July 2019